Style Feed

Style Feed

William
Oliver

The World's Top Fashion Blogs

Selected by
Susie Bubble

Prestel

Munich · London · New York

Contents:
Blogs by Date Started

Foreword   6
Introduction   14

2011
The Coveteur   18

2010
The Man Repeller   28
Industrie   36
Anna Dello Russo   44

2009
Fred Butler Style   52
Hanneli   60
Patternity   68
The Blonde Salad   76
Stop It Right Now   82
What Katie Wore   88
Cocorosa   96

2008
Style Rookie   104
Advanced Style   112
The Dandy Project   118
Jak & Jil   124
Lulu and Your Mom   132
Hapsical   138
Karla's Closet   146
Luxirare   152
Dapper Kid   158
Vanessa Jackman   164
Park & Cube   172
Buckets and Spades   180

2007

Disneyrollergirl   188
Kate Loves Me   196
The Business of Fashion   204
Fashionista   210
Amlul   218
Style Salvage   226
Selectism   234

2006

Un Nouveau Ideal   242
Kingdom of Style   250
Face Hunter   258
Garance Doré   266
StyleClicker   274
Stil in Berlin   280
Street Peeper   288
Style Bubble   296

2005

Hypebeast   306
A Shaded View on Fashion   312

Acknowledgements   318
Picture Credits   319

Foreword

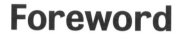

Susie Bubble

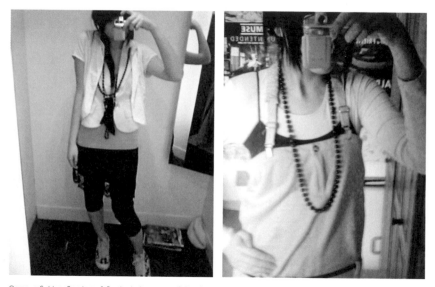

Some of the first self-shot images of Susie ever to appear online,
posted on The Fashion Spot forum in 2005

I had a dirty habit from 2005 to 2006, coinciding neatly with my final year of studying history at University College London, when I was slightly terrified of what graduating would actually mean. Every day I would escape from lectures and seminars and log on to The Fashion Spot, a community forum where fashion lovers and industry insiders could pore over collections, models, magazine editorials and personal style. I succumbed to having a second life on the Internet, chatting to people I had never met in person and sharing parts of my life with strangers long before the explosion of Facebook and Twitter.

The Fashion Spot was also where I first discovered the act of sharing your personal style, something that would rapidly spiral into today's phenomenon of fashion blogging. I'd take a picture of my outfit in the mirror, palms sweating, because it seemed such a preposterous act of narcissism at the time. A quick upload (without the now-standard Photoshop clean-up process) and my self-image would be out there for members to bestow virtual karma points and encouraging comments on. The Fashion Spot was in effect the gestating cocoon for the beginnings of my own fashion blog and arguably the start of fashion blogging's explosion.

When I finally did graduate, the progression to starting an actual fashion blog was natural. In March 2006 Style Bubble went live quietly. I set out with a mission statement: I didn't want to rehash *Women's Wear Daily* news bites, I admitted I wasn't a fashion insider, I said I had peculiar and particular tastes and I acknowledged that I could only write about what I know and love. In hindsight, outsiders would see this as a tactical move into self-publishing but initially I didn't view Style Bubble as a media outlet. It was more of a hobby I could indulge in, a place where I could explore my own taste in fashion. It is that feeling of exploration, together with discovery, that – although Style Bubble has now become a full-time endeavour – I hope to emulate today.

The addiction to blogging was, and is, something of a guilty pleasure. At first there were few others that I knew in real life who could understand what it felt like to rush home and geekily offload pictures from an exhibition or visit to an exciting store, or share a new designer discovery with readers. Only through following links of comments on the blog did I find myself a few allies. I count the likes of Michelle from Scottish fashion blog Kingdom of Style as an early cohort who could sympathize with the trials and tribulations, as well as the joys, that came with fashion blogging.

Not all blogs are created equal and it was precisely the multitude of differences that made it so exciting. When I first happened upon Style Rookie, a blog written by a then 12-year-old girl called Tavi Gevinson, it blew me away to read such a kindred and unique voice coming from a bedroom in the suburbs of Chicago. It's no surprise that Gevinson has gone on to become an editor in her own right, with the successful teen-focused web magazine *Rookie*, an unimaginable feat when I first started blogging.

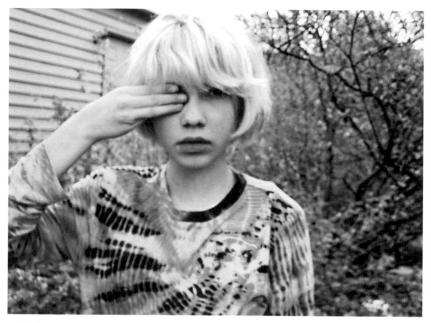

Style Rookie

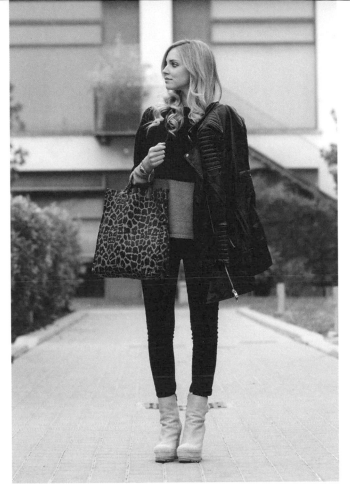

The Blonde Salad

As the platform began to grow in popularity, sub-categories emerged under the umbrella term 'fashion blogs'. There are personal style bloggers like The Blonde Salad, Amlul and Hanneli, who constantly share photos documenting their own clothing and, in part, lifestyle. This has subsequently led to celebrity status for a number of these authors, garnering them opportunities to collaborate with high-end fashion brands as models, spokespeople and, in some cases, designers.

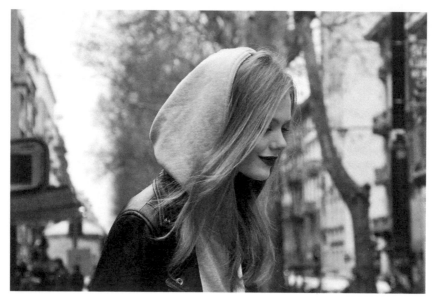

Jak & Jil

There are street style bloggers for whom blogging is a vehicle to showcase their photography and their ability to capture a particular zeitgeist on the streets, at parties and, more recently, outside numerous international fashion week shows. Tommy Ton of Jak & Jil and Phil Oh of Street Peeper, for example, have become official street style photographers for Style.com and American *Vogue*'s website respectively. This is a notable act of official sanction by the fashion media establishment and has placed these blogger/photographers in a class of their own.

Then there are blogs that can be recognized as fully fledged websites or media outlets. They have infrastructures resembling those of print publications, but the content unabashedly sticks to their cornered niche. They have become well-respected sources of information for the industry and beyond, be it the latest in streetwear and menswear on Hypebeast, a light-hearted take on news on Fashionista, or detailed analysis of the industry on The Business of Fashion.

Finally, there is a string of indefinable but defiantly recognizable voices who comment on fashion in their own specific ways, from Luxirare's incredible photography of mind-boggling DIY projects and food creations to Patternity's clever observations of patterns that impact all design spectra. There's also the more recent phenomenon of traditional print editors, such as Anna Dello Russo, editor-at-large of *Vogue Nippon*, turning to blogging as a form of personal expression and an extension of their own brands.

What I and all these other fashion bloggers discovered early on was the simultaneous power and vulnerability of putting yourself out there. My first negative criticism was something along the lines of 'You're not a journalist. You're not a stylist. Stick to what you know.' Wasn't that the appeal of fashion blogs? It's a criticism that has been levelled against bloggers since the beginning and continues to dog us. Questions of whether blogging is a passing fad or will threaten the existence of print magazines are common. The answer to both is currently a resounding no. Fashion bloggers haven't blipped into a Web 2.0 black hole and don't look like they will be going away any time soon. Magazines, especially those with a strongly independent identity or niche readership, are still going strong.

Street Peeper

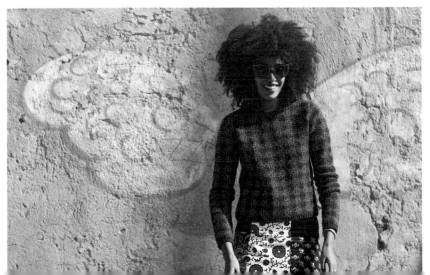

There seems to be a growing appreciation for taking in information at multiple speeds – slowly through style biannuals and monthly magazines and quickly through RSS feeds and browser bookmarks. Print and online publications can and do now co-exist, and blogs cross-pollinate with sanctioned fashion media outlets. Mainstream fashion publications feature bloggers or ask them to write columns, do guest styling or adopt the format of a street style blog, photographing clothes on non-models. Fashion PR agencies and brands have begun to tackle the question of how to deal with bloggers in their own marketing strategies. This is a reverberating recognition of bloggers as more than just renegades that will disappear and has resulted in many high-profile brand-blogger alliances.

In response to this collaboration between brands and bloggers, the professionalism of the platform has been scrutinized with ongoing fascination. After 'What is the future of fashion blogging?', 'How do you make money?' is the question I get asked the most, and is something that I personally don't mind tackling. If you see an ad on my blog, it's there because it's paying my rent. For me, these questions actually skirt the main issue at hand, which is the content of the fashion blog itself.

The bottom line should be: are we still enjoying what bloggers do? The preoccupation with how professional, influential and financially well-off a fashion blogger is can make people lose sight of what makes fashion blogs such a fascinating source of inspiration. As a blogger myself, I have to keep asking whether I still have my original passion and whether it still shows in the content. Relishing the freedom over what you blog is an important part of that. As soon as it becomes a chore, it starts to show in the quality of the writing.

When I started the blog, I tagged it with the line 'I'm a fashion outsider.' People will say this proclamation doesn't stand true anymore, but I like to think that maintaining perspective helps make me grateful for everything that Style Bubble has become. I still sit at fashion shows wondering whether a PR will suddenly ask me to leave. It's savouring that newness and seeing things

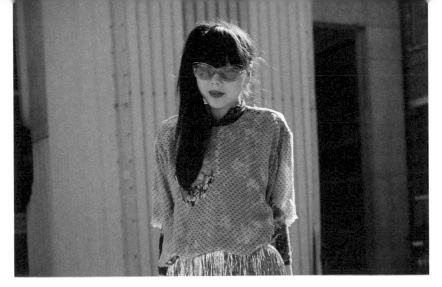
Susie now

in an unjaded light that spurs me on, and it is that untainted
point of view that captures readers' imaginations.

As a reader and observer of fashion blogs, it's still about
unearthing captivating sources to latch on to as new daily
reads. There are hundreds of thousands of fashion blogs and
there's no denying there are plenty that are bad. A strong
and distinctive identity has never felt more essential. For
me, the most interesting voices and points of view do not
necessarily come from blogs with 5 million monthly page views.

I joined the fashion blogging party in 2006, awkwardly
shuffling my feet with a cup of punch. Over the years the party
may have become increasingly busy, but the simultaneously good
and bad thing about blogging is that everybody is invited. The
blogs we have selected here represent the best of who is at that
party, but that isn't to say it is a definitive list of the most
influential blogs or those with the biggest readership. *Style Feed*
isn't a hard-line ranking system, but a celebration of blogs we
feel have longevity as valid voices in the ever-noisy world of the
fashion media, and as inspirational forces to be reckoned with.

Introduction

Though style blogging has had a relatively short lifespan,
it has rapidly developed from a series of disconnected online
fanzines to become an integral part of the fashion business.
Today it is easy to take their impact for granted but, in the
beginning, bloggers were not always welcomed by some of the
industry insiders they so admired.

Fashion is built on desirability and aspiration; on the creation
of beautiful objects that people strive to obtain in order
to enhance how they look, feel and present themselves to others.
Brands are strictly managed and correct representation is key,
with journalists, stylists and editors often working under rigid
guidelines. To some extent, blogging shattered this notion. As
unmoderated, independent voices, bloggers had the freedom to say
whatever they wanted about the style, quality or relevance of any
fashion 'product' they chose. They also had the ability to reach
virtually anyone, anywhere.

At first, the fashion industry found blogging difficult
to understand. Gradually, though, blogs established themselves
as truly personal takes on style and their importance was
recognized. They may offer different perspectives on fashion
to the ones we are historically used to, but they highlight
the excitement felt by real people who actually wear, or want
to wear, the clothes featured. Over time this has become valued
by brands and designers who regularly work with bloggers in
a variety of ways, from collaborations on bags, shoes and clothes
to using them as models and ambassadors, with the lucky few
sitting front-row at catwalk shows.

While blogging may at one time have been seen as a passing
fad, today it is not uncommon for high-profile blogs to reach
an audience of 25,000 people a day. It is all too easy, though,
to be wowed by the vast number of people that one blogger,
often working from their own home, can reach and subsequently
to put too much emphasis on the commercial effect they might
have. What is important to remember is that at its root, fashion
blogging is born out of an honest passion for clothing design.
And, for some, blogging has become not only a way of commentating
and discussing, but also contributing.

Blogs can be highly creative visual experiments, diaries
or resources and it is this aspect that shone through while
putting together this book. Everyone featured and interviewed
here has taken the idea of what blogging is somewhere new,
whether they have a unique approach or a strong aesthetic
sensibility, or are doing something that is genuinely inspiring
and intriguing. Ultimately *Style Feed* is exactly as described
on the cover: the world's top fashion blogs, whatever form they
may take.

William Oliver

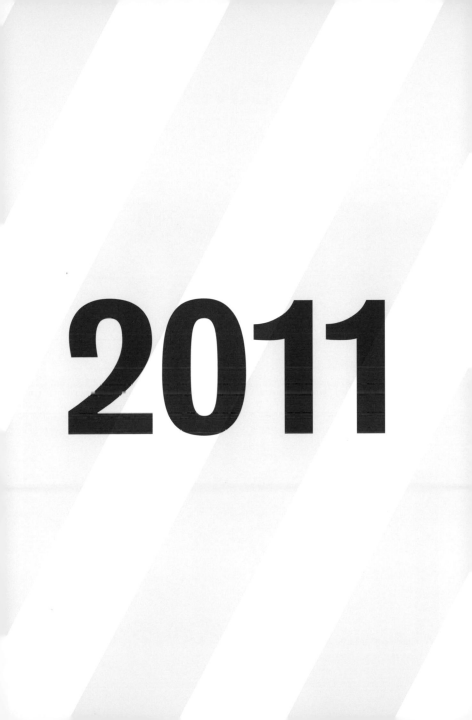

2011

The Coveteur

Erin Kleinberg & Stephanie Mark
Photography by Jake Rosenberg
thecoveteur.com

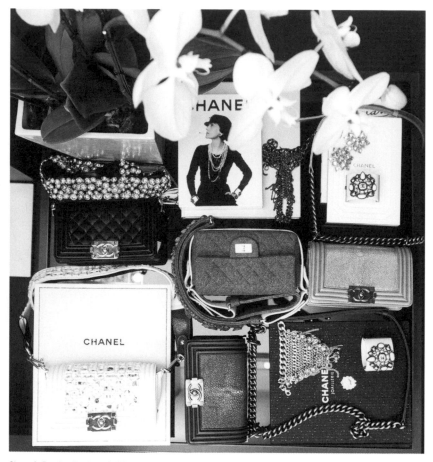

Chanel Paris-Bombay Collection, Métiers d'Art. Paris

Though it's only been up and running since 2011, The Coveteur has already firmly established itself as a high-profile fashion blog. One of the most innovative examples of what can be done with the platform, the site provides an intimate view into the style values of notable scenesters, including Anna Dello Russo, Khloe Kardashian, Rachel Zoe, Simon Doonan and Jonathan Adler. Set up by stylists Erin Kleinberg and Stephanie Mark, with photography by Jake Rosenberg, it pulls together all three contributors' creative backgrounds to produce intriguing content that goes beyond the industry facade. Using contacts established through their commercial styling careers, Mark and Kleinberg have garnered incredible access to the homes, handbags and closets of the fashion elite, artfully arranging and photographing what they find. Collaborations with Chanel, WhoWhatWear, Rachel Zoe and New York Fashion Week have all cemented the project's respectability, as has being voted Blog of the Year by leading e-commerce site Net-A-Porter.

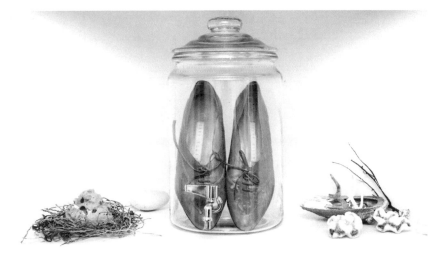

Jeff Halmos and Lisa Mayock. Co-founder, Shipley & Halmos; co-founder, Vena Cava. New York

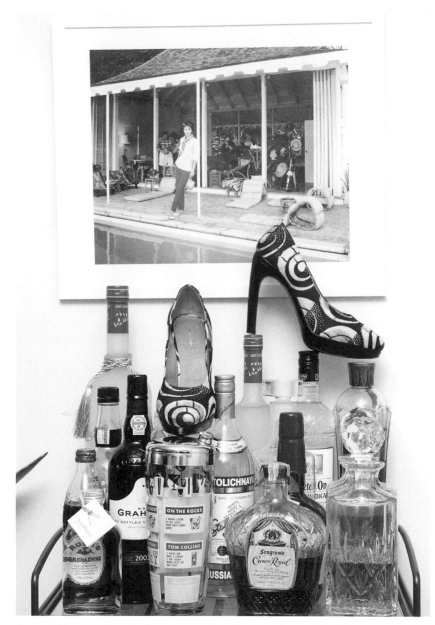

Joanna Hillman, senior fashion market editor, *Harper's Bazaar*. New York

Erin Kleinberg & Stephanie Mark

'We saw a void in the industry and that's really
what it's all about – finding little cracks that
need to be filled. We wanted to deconstruct the
idea of street style and take it one step further
and go behind the scenes – to show people how
the tastemakers they have become obsessed with
as a result of street style blogs get dressed every
day, and to deconstruct their sartorial choices.
We're always inspired by our subject's style, home
or career; we really seek to showcase people who
are influential in today's culture and will have
a lasting impact in decades to come. There's always
more to a person than meets the eye and we take
pride in really getting to know our subjects.
The anecdotes we get from them give our readers
greater insight into who the person is and where
they come from.

Our aesthetic is sleek, clean and modern;
one of our major points of differentiation
was establishing a site devoid of advertisers.
We really wanted our readers to come to the
site and not be bombarded with pop-ups and
banners that took away from our exclusive
content. The blogosphere is oversaturated
with a sea of sameness but we're dedicated to
providing readers with images and information
that they're not going to be able to find
elsewhere. When we go inside someone's home,
it's not about showcasing that "It" bag or
pair of shoes that every street style blog
has snapped – it's about showcasing a person's
style by curating individual pieces.'

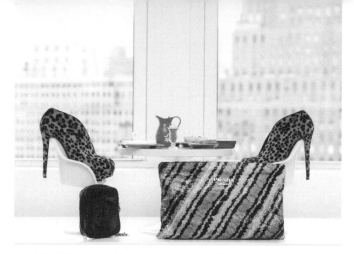

Jennifer Fisher, jewellery designer, Jennifer Fisher Jewelry; outerwear designer, Wyler. New York

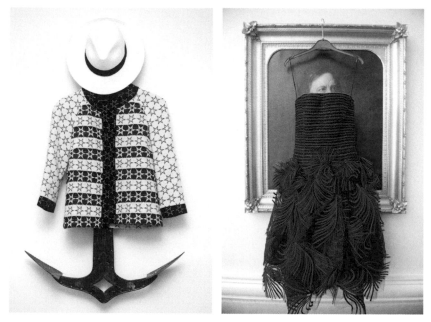

Left: Joanna Hillman
Right: Dee Dee Taylor Eustace, architect and interior designer, Taylor Hannah Architect Inc. Toronto

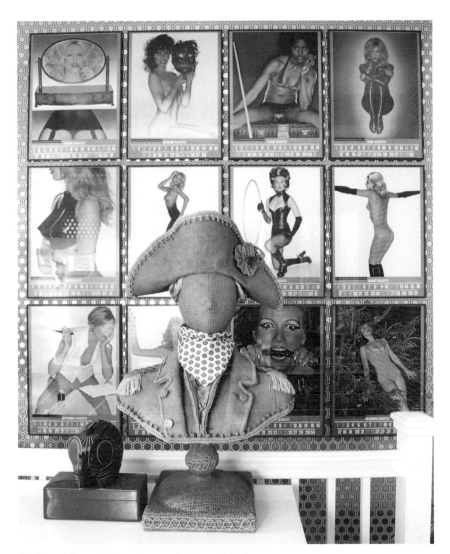

Jonathan Adler and Simon Doonan. Potter and designer;
creative ambassador-at-large, Barneys New York. New York

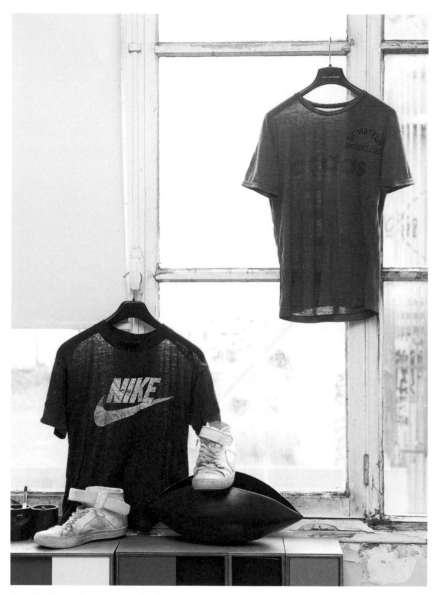

Jerome Dreyfuss, designer. Paris

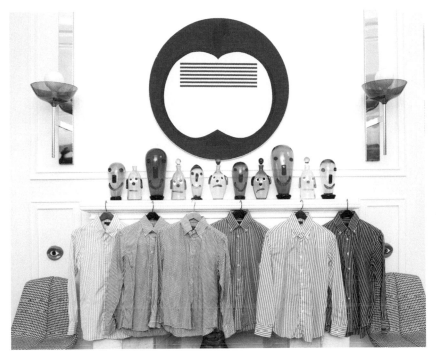

Jonathan Adler and Simon Doonan

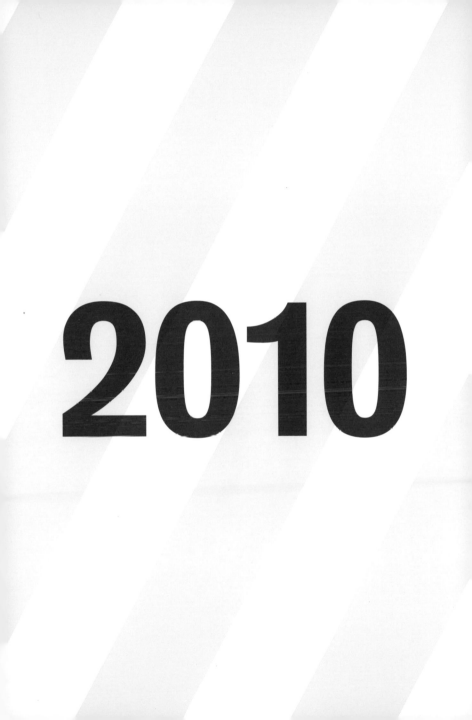

The Man Repeller

Leandra Medine

manrepeller.com

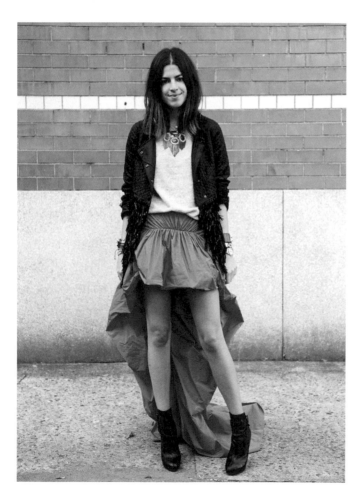

Originator of the terms 'arm party' for an extensive collection of bracelets worn at once, and 'man-repelling', defined on the blog itself as 'outfitting oneself in a sartorially offensive way that will result in repelling members of the opposite sex', Leandra Medine's The Man Repeller is a witty read. One part social commentary on the collision between male and female tastes and one part personal style guide, Medine's blog combines sharply written content with a deep appreciation for fashion. A journalism graduate, the New York-based Medine has previously written for publications including *New York Magazine* and *Harper's Bazaar* as well as interning at Valentino and Phillip Lim. Her tongue-in-cheek humour and celebration of harem trousers, denim overalls and all things man-repelling have earned her both a loyal following and a good reputation in the fashion industry. In the first two years of her blogging career she collaborated on films with Michael Kors, Prabal Gurung and Simon Doonan, received a profile in the *New York Times* and secured her own book project, pencilled for 2013.

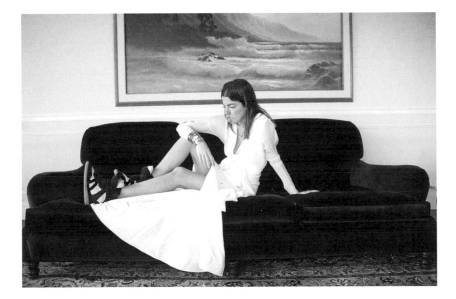

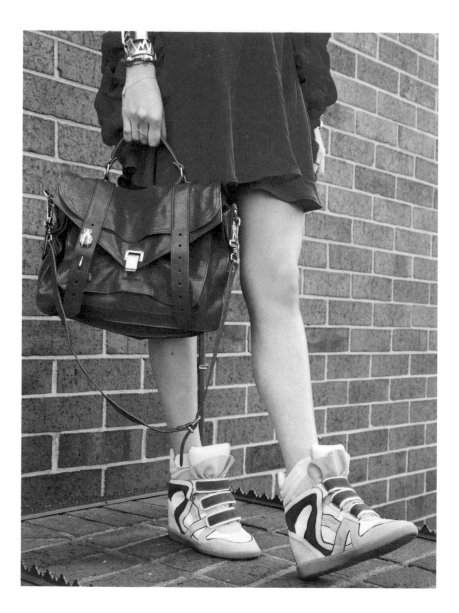

Leandra Medine

'I was lucky to found The Man Repeller on the brink of changing times, when blogging was transitioning from hobby to sustainable career. When I wrote for publications I found that my work was edited too much and it lost the quirk and charm that I thought strung it together. By blogging I was able to publish whatever I wanted, maintain final say and be my own editor, which is a special thing. My blog started as a pretty simple "Would this repel men or not?" Now it's more about questioning whether or not what I'm featuring is both aesthetically pleasing and wearable art.

Initially, The Man Repeller was a commentary on culture. I wasn't the man-repeller; I was just making the observations. Over time, I started putting images of myself on the site, sort of took on this role and created a persona. It has expanded from just women's fashion being repulsive to men to women consciously dressing for themselves and almost hoping that they will in fact achieve man-repeller status.

For me, fashion blogging brings an element of realness. The girls that read magazines and want to change the industry finally have an opportunity to leave a footprint and have their voices heard.'

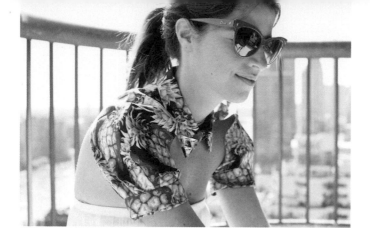

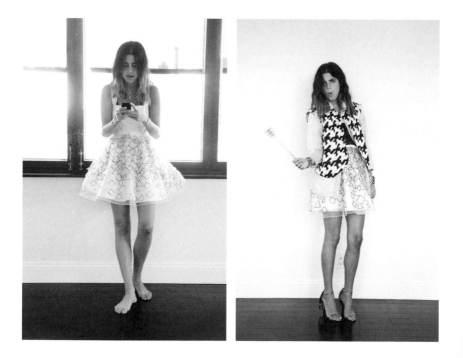

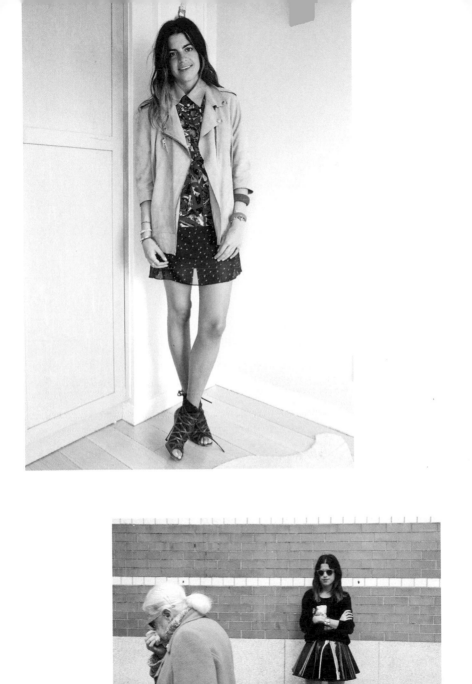

33

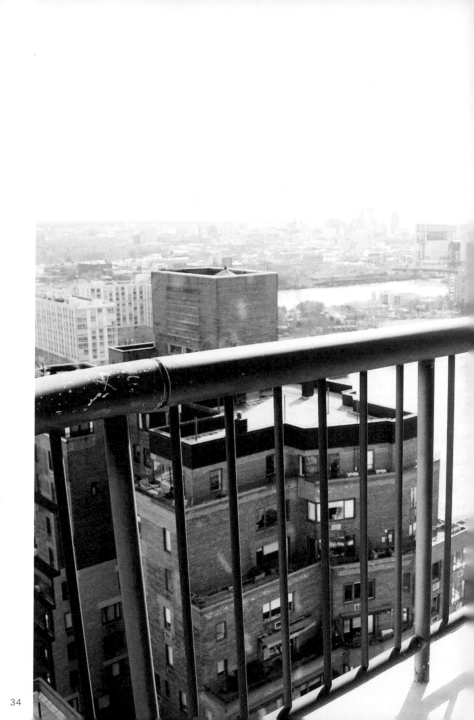

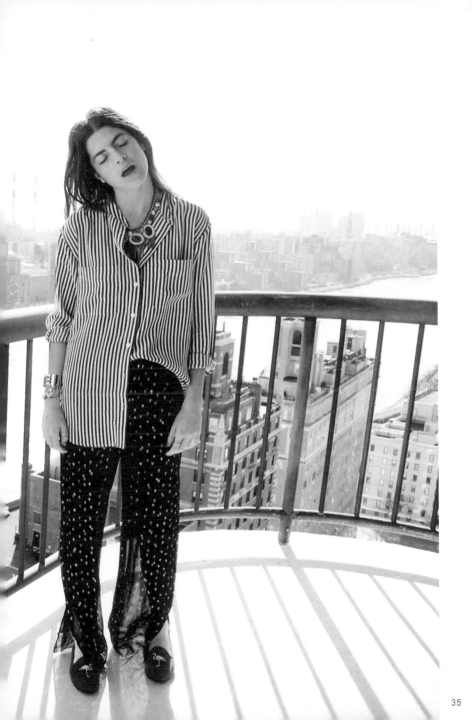

Industrie

Erik Torstensson & Jens Grede

industrie.nowmanifest.com

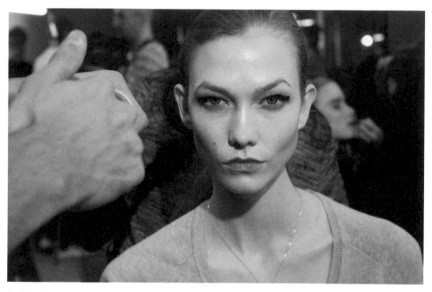

Karlie Kloss at Paris Fashion Week: Kenzo 2012

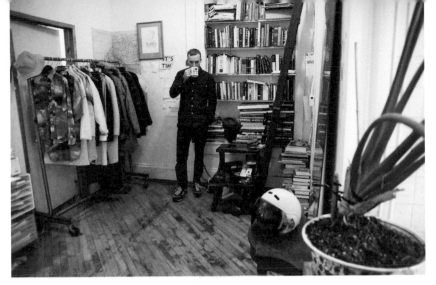

At Patrik Ervell's studio, New York City

After working for Tyler Brûlé's *Wallpaper**, setting up
advertising and creative agency Saturday and publishing *Man
About Town* magazine, London-based duo Erik Torstensson and
Jens Grede decided to launch *Industrie* magazine in 2009. Focused
solely on the people behind the scenes of the fashion industry –
photographers, stylists, editors and designers themselves rather
than the collections they produce – the magazine is based around
unrivalled access to its subjects. *Industrie* ventures into
homes and workplaces to look at creative practices, provides
opinions on the industry and how it is changing and features
conversations with people from celebrities to models and those
in the know. A natural progression from the magazine was the
blog of the same name, which they founded the following year.
The online *Industrie* site avoids the type of in-depth, analytical
interviews and features found in the printed version and
provides 'something snappier and a little more easygoing'.

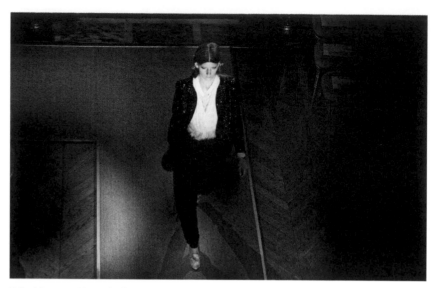

Valentino run-through, Paris

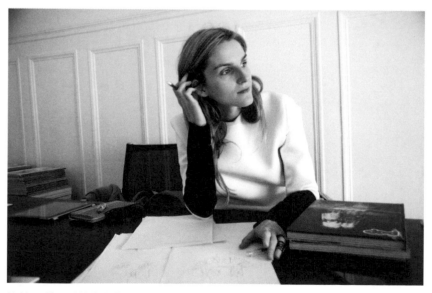

At the office with Gaia Repossi

Erik Torstensson & Jens Grede

'We started the blog because we wanted people
to read the content we produce regardless of where
they live and, perhaps more importantly, because
not all content is right for a printed magazine.
In print we prefer more in-depth, longer pieces and
photography and on the blog we can try new formats.
We love content, regardless of how it is published.
Our aesthetic is simple, elegant and considered,
straight to the point. We go by gut feeling. Are
we excited by this today? We also love things that
are amazing but might have been forgotten. We don't
report on other people's events; we create our own
original content. It is a magazine in blog form.
This was only made possible because of our network
of incredible collaborators. They see and live what
we feature.'

At New York Fashion Week: Lindsey Wixson

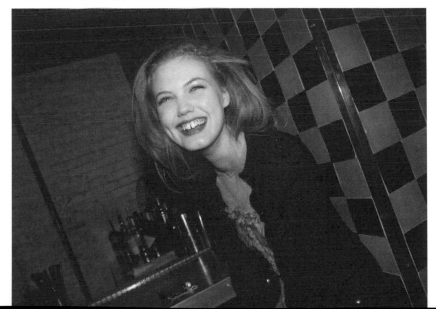

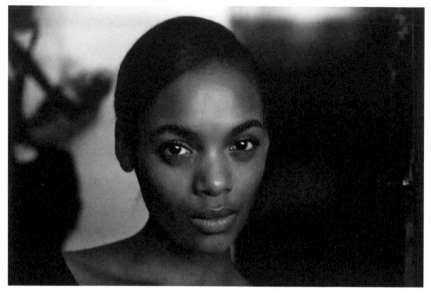

At Paris Fashion Week: Dries Van Noten 2012

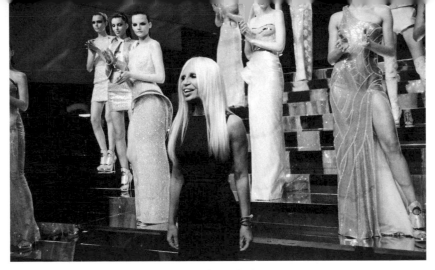

Donatella Versace at the Atelier Versace Show, Paris

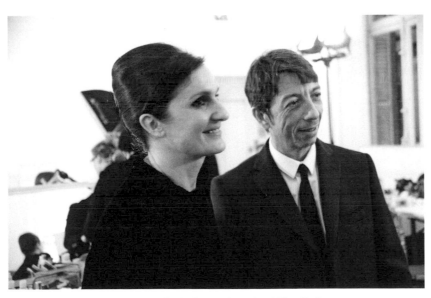

Valentino's creative directors, Maria Grazia Chiuri and Pier Paolo
Piccioli, backstage at Couture Fashion Week, Paris
Overleaf: At Paris Fashion Week: Kenzo 2012

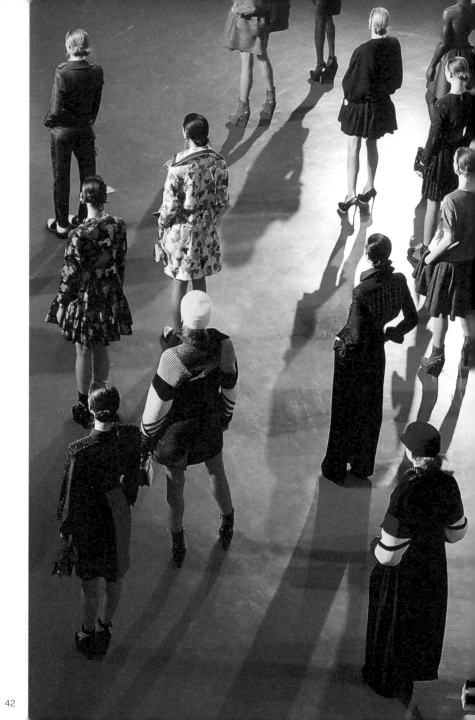

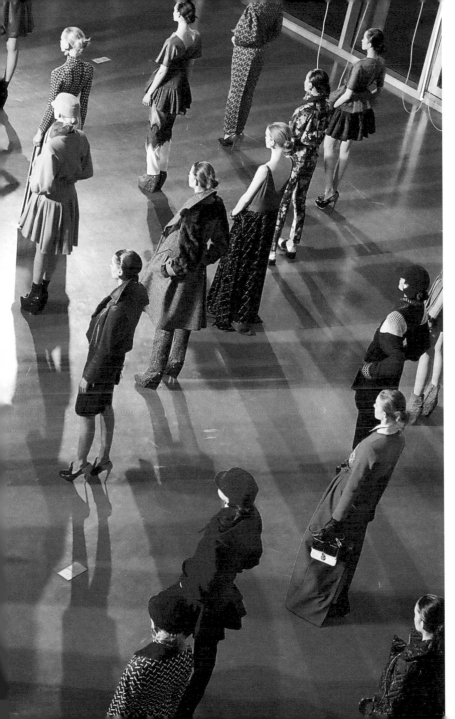

Anna Dello Russo

Anna Dello Russo
annadellorusso.com

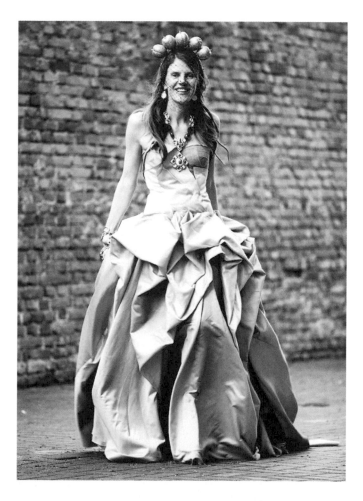

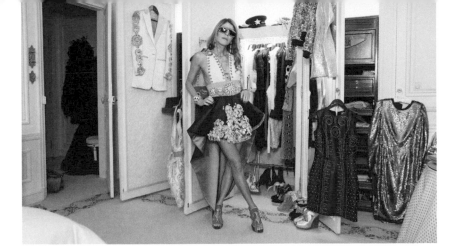

A true industry insider who has spent almost 20 years under the roof of international publishing house Condé Nast, Anna Dello Russo had already amassed impressive fashion world credentials before starting her life as a leading blogger. She has worked as the fashion editor of *Vogue Italia* and the editor of *L'Uomo Vogue* and is currently fashion director and editor-at-large of *Vogue Nippon*. Although firmly established within her own generation, in 2010 Dello Russo wanted to connect to a younger audience and, after noticing what was happening with the online social world, felt blogging would be the ideal vehicle. Since starting her site, now notorious for its glamorous, vivacious and high-octane aesthetic, Dello Russo has accrued a huge international fan base looking for an insight into her luxurious and beautiful world. Her diary-like posts often focus on images of Anna sporting a variety of colourful, chic and playful looks, consistently teamed with her signature superb shoes, taken from her personal collection of over 4,000 pairs. She has become one of the most recognized members of the upper echelons of the blogging community, with her appearance and outfits at various events worldwide documented avidly by an army of street style photographers. Alongside her attendance at fashion shows and parties, the blog also features beautiful pieces of clothing, objects or people she has met, each chosen to inspire experimental creativity in her readers.

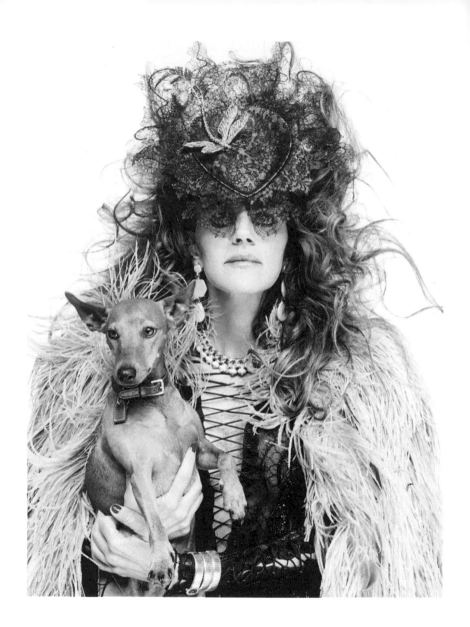

Anna Dello Russo

'When you feel uncomfortable with something, you should work at it. This is what I have learnt from yoga. If you try a pose and it is easy then it doesn't make sense to keep on with it; you should do the opposite. When I find something difficult, I work at it to find familiarity. In the beginning, I forced myself to gain confidence with blogging because I didn't want to be in this mobile world, with my computer still attached to the wall. I wanted to be part of this new process and show the "behind-the-scenes" fashion world. For me, blogging is about getting in touch with a new generation, with an audience younger than me. I keep my blog almost like a teenage diary, but the concept is deeper. Blogging is a playground, experimental but always joyful, and I wanted to be creative with the new media, which is why I decorate my posts and images. When I am working with an assistant I always tell them that beauty is all around you in life, but it is about how you edit it. Blogging is organic, like planting a seed. You start it off, but then it grows in its own way. It follows the light, feels the love and changes every day. My blog has given me more visibility and opened me up to people around the world. It has made me feel less stiff, more approachable. It has led people to think about me differently and allowed me to get involved in many different projects. My blog is my laboratory and it has opened up so many opportunities.'

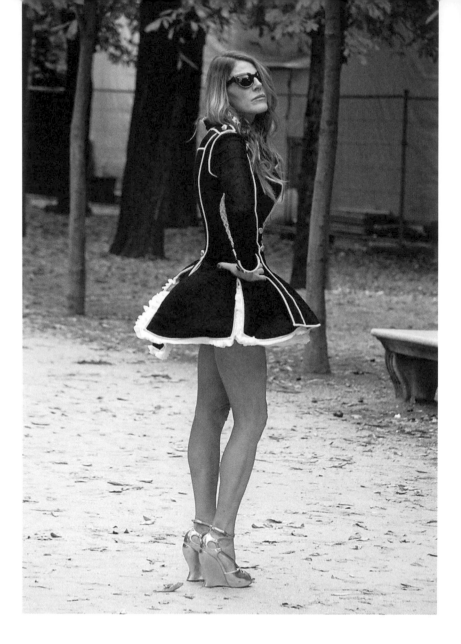

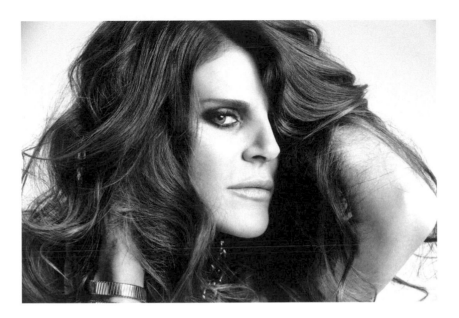

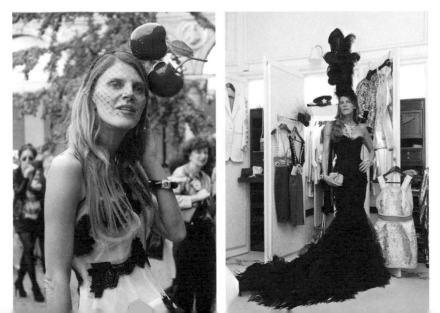

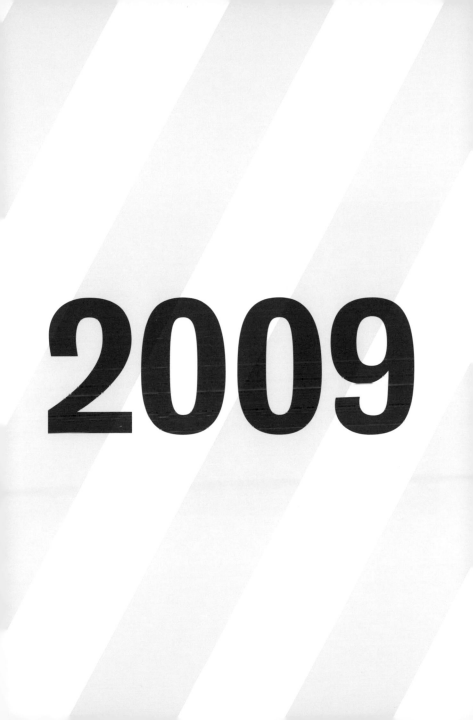

2009

Fred Butler Style

Fred Butler

fredbutlerstyle.blogspot.co.uk

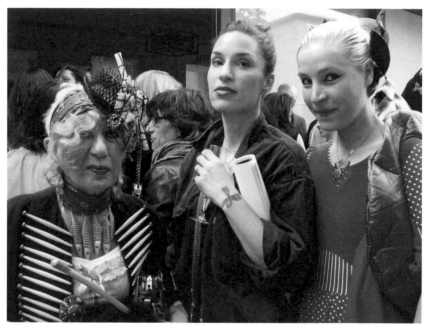

L to R: Anna Piaggi, Elisha Smith-Leverock, Fred Butler

Starting out as an accessories and set designer, Londoner Fred Butler established herself as a firm fixture in the fashion industry through her constant and uninhibited passion for colour and pattern. Fred Butler Style, which she set up in 2009, gave her a chance to document the world around her and is, as she describes it, 'an instant diary and record of my busy life'. The blog posts mainly focus on projects she has an interest in or is working on, or on people she meets and finds inspiring. After garnering a wide group of collaborators and fans, Butler presented her first full womenswear collection as part of New Gen at London Fashion Week in 2008 for Autumn/Winter 2009 and has shown each season since. Her work has been featured in numerous style publications, with her accessories and props incorporated into forward-thinking editorials for the likes of *Dazed & Confused*, *AnOther Magazine*, the *Style* section of the *Sunday Times* and *Wonderland*. She has also constructed pieces for musicians including Nicki Minaj, Man Like Me and Patrick Wolf as well as creating Lady Gaga's iconic 'Telephone' headpiece.

Rosy Nicholas in her studio

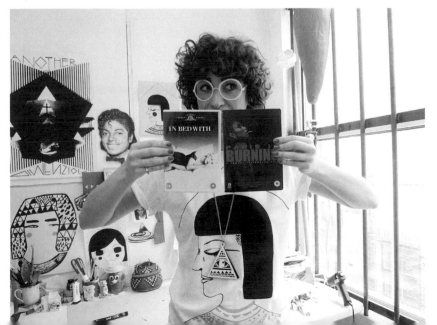

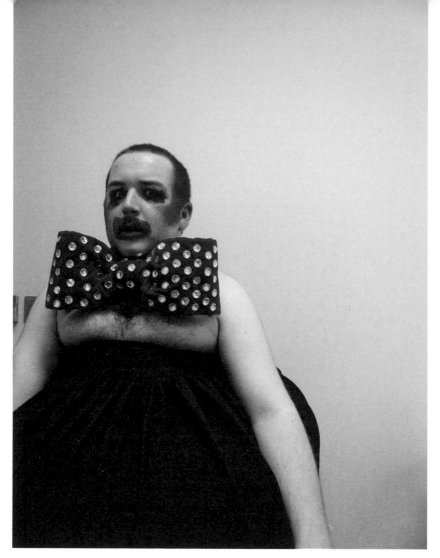

Scottee at The Brit Awards aftershow party

Fred Butler

'I love historical works that have captured
a chapter in time as a cultural resource, such
as Maripol's Polaroids of New York City or
Peter Schlesinger's photography of Hockney and
his incredible clique. It's so lucky that these
everyday scenarios were documented and I was
aware that I myself was in a fascinating situation
by living and working at the epicentre of the arts
in London. I'm a believer in sharing information
for the greater good, so I wanted to expose all
the emerging talent surrounding me and spread
that privileged information.

My blog reflects my idiosyncratic tastes and
aesthetics: colour, colour, colour with a graphic
undertone and a slant for themes that combine both
futuristic insight and retro nostalgia. Clothes,
artwork, jewellery: whatever it is, it has to pop
off the screen and be instantly clear and alive.

I get excited about discovering artists who
are into the same stimuli as myself. I want to
promote positivity via an uplifting perspective
with fresh, alternative ideas to the safe and
repetitive reportage in the mainstream press. It's
led to establishing many unexpected and fantastic
friendships which I treasure greatly and still
can't believe, but it does mean that I never have
one minute of free time. I'm constantly researching
new articles and keeping up to date with previous
featured stories to stay in touch with the latest
developments. I have to take time out of my own
design work, but it's like a brilliant book I can't
put down. Blogs can be neutral and untainted
and provide pure perception, which is why they
have become an unprecedented success story. It's
democracy that is the key.'

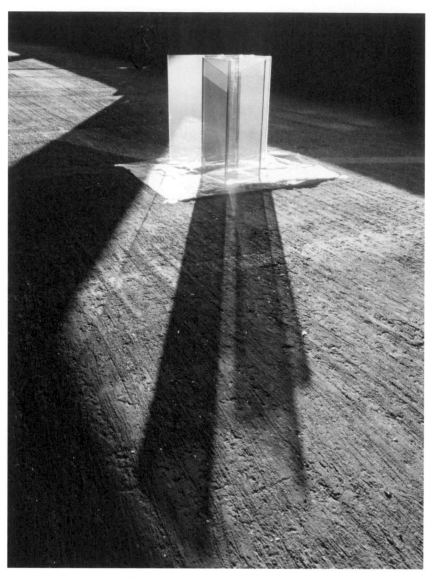

Samuel Nias piece at Bold Tendencies

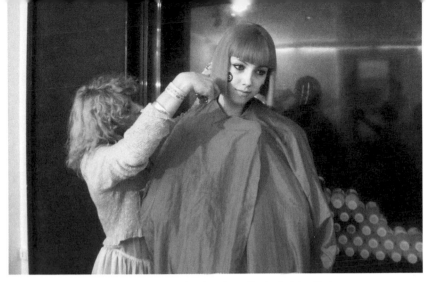

Lyndell Mansfield backstage at Zandra Rhodes show, Paris Fashion Week

Beth Ditto at Lovebox Festival

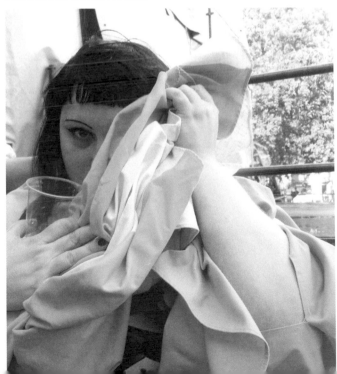

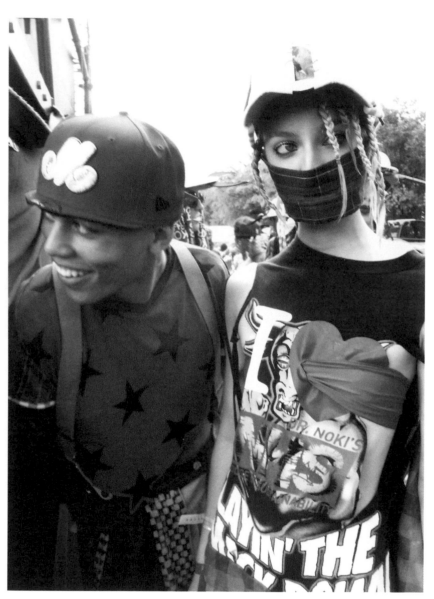

Dudley O'Shaughnessy modelling for NOKI

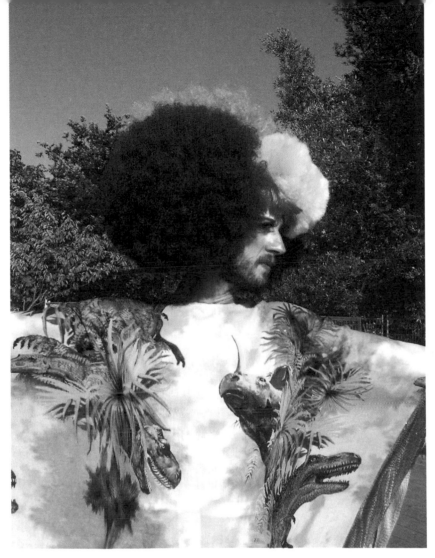

Jonny Woo

Hanneli

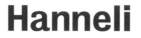

Hanneli Mustaparta

hanneli.com

Hanneli: Greene Street, New York City

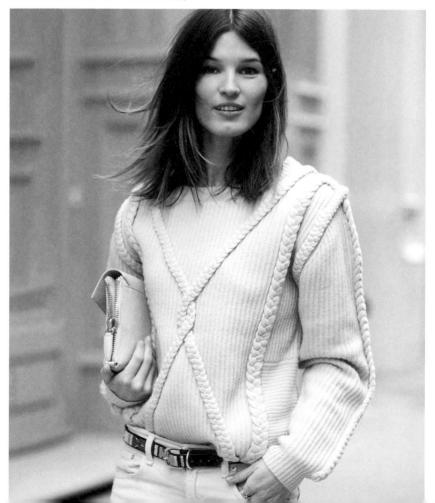

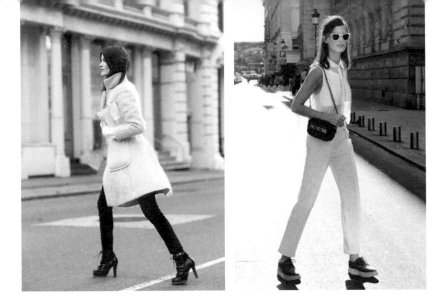

After being spotted at the age of 17 by photographer Per Heimly, Norwegian-born, New York-based Hanneli Mustaparta started her career as a model, working for eight years internationally. In 2009 she started her blog, for which she used her previously lesser-known skills as a photographer to capture the people, clothes and places that inspired her. Focusing initially on street style, her beautiful, classic images have become renowned for their chic feel and her fantastic access to the industry. Mustaparta has photographed everyone from Stefano Pilati and Arizona Muse to Lindsey Wixson and presents these images alongside self-portraits. Now shooting for Vogue.com, styling for H&M, co-hosting CBS's webcast 'Fashion's Night Out' and working on a t-shirt collaboration with Zara, Mustaparta has gone from her blog to numerous other projects and broadened what was once a hobby into a full-time career.

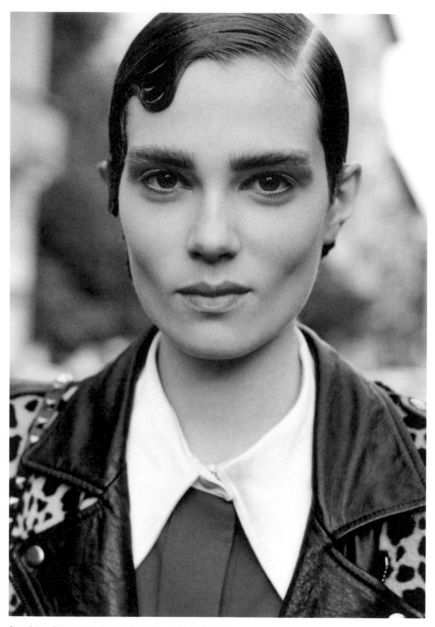

Caroline Brasch Nielsen after Prada's S/S 11 show

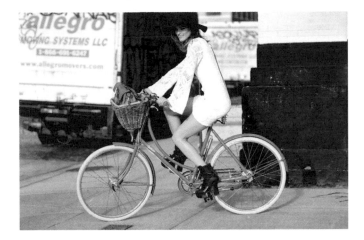

Hanneli Mustaparta

'I've always been interested in photography
and have taken a lot of pictures over the years.
At some point I decided that I wanted to do
something with my favourite shots instead of just
keeping them in folders in my laptop. I initially
wanted to focus on the style of other people and
on editorials that I loved, but there was a time,
particularly between fashion weeks, when it was
very quiet and I would struggle to find anyone on
the streets of New York whom I wanted to photograph
for the blog - it was freezing and people were
bundled up. My solution was to shoot myself in
outfits I loved in order to have some content. That
evolved into putting all my inspirations on to the
blog and now being in a position where I am able
to inspire readers all over the world.

I am intrigued by things that feel fresh, new and
different. I like things looking clean with a twist.
I love things that are unexpected yet structured.'

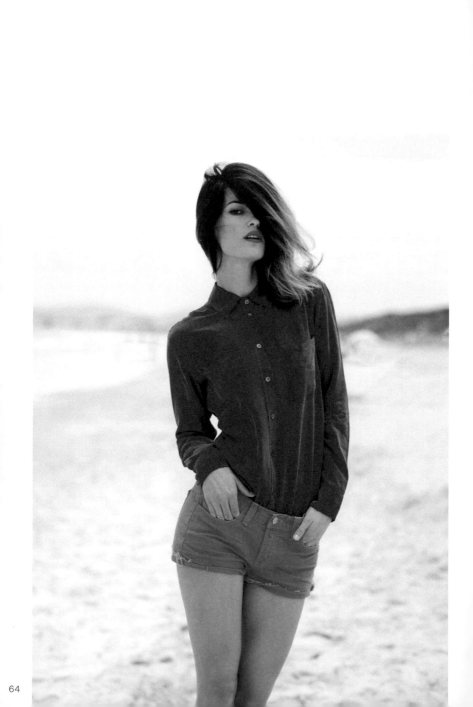

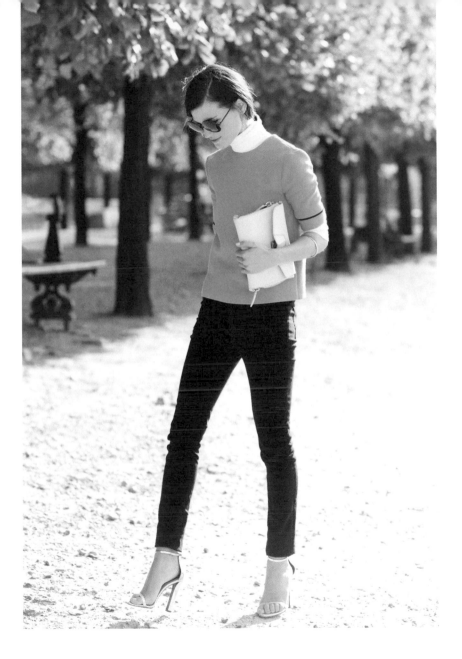

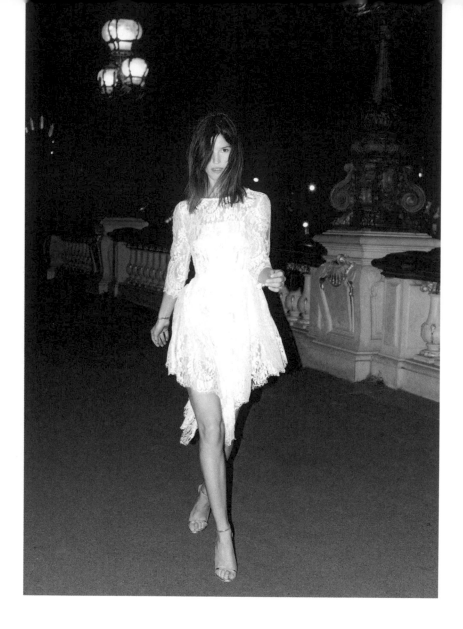

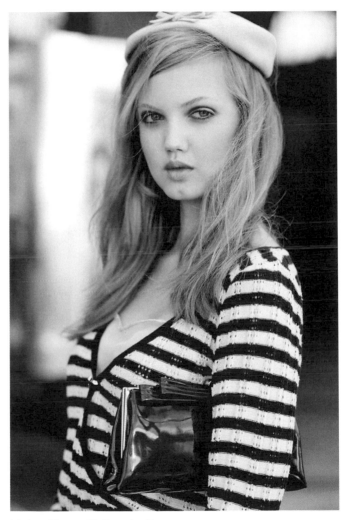

Lindsey Wixson off the catwalk

Patternity

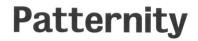

Anna Murray & Grace Winteringham

patternity.co.uk

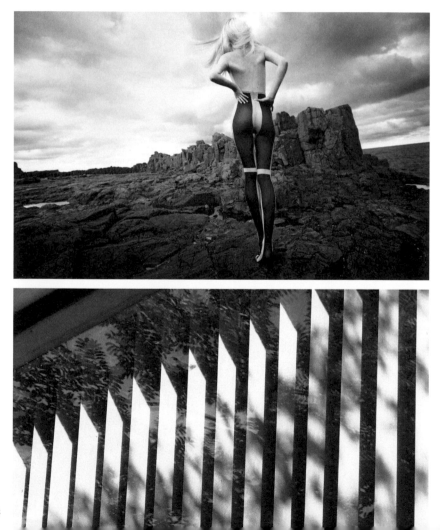

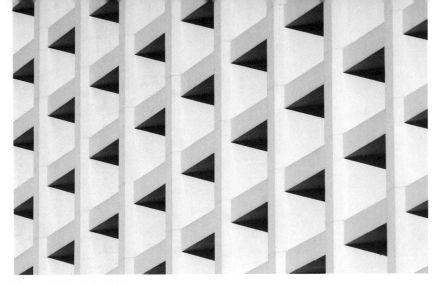

Above: Murray triangles
Opposite top: Block Out Rock Out Tights
Opposite bottom: Aqua angles

Londoners Anna Murray and Grace Winteringham have a plethora
of fashion industry experience behind them. Murray has worked
with Louis Vuitton, Selfridges and Mulberry as an art director
since graduating in 2006 while Winteringham has collaborated
with Alexander McQueen and Tom Dixon as a freelance textiles
designer. Meeting by chance through their work, their
shared love of pattern brought them together. While they come
from differing career backgrounds, Patternity was born out
of a desire to share their aesthetic. Part resource and
inspiration, part musings, the blog has gained a wide realm
of readers (including the likes of designer Phoebe Philo from
Céline) who come to Patternity for its unique observations.
The blog records the patterns that its founders see all around
them, whether in buildings, leaves, tangled wires or clothes
themselves. In 2011 *Wallpaper** magazine voted theirs the sixth
best site on the web out of a shortlist of 20. Also operating
as a design studio, the duo have embarked on a number of
collaborations and have embedded themselves firmly in London's
design community.

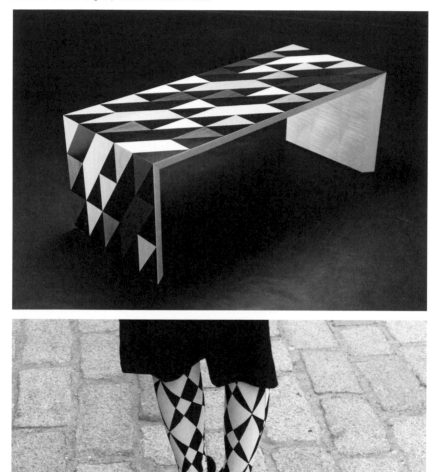

Anna Murray & Grace Winteringham

'Patternity is about the putting together
of patterns and seeing visual coincidences from
one image to the next. Though we love the natural
world and the patterns it contains, we tend
to veer toward a stronger, bolder, often quite
masculine and manmade look, with a focus on urban
environments and constructed forms. Patternity
essentially began long before our site was set
up. It was an idea that came about through a shared
way of seeing the world despite our seemingly
different backgrounds. Upon meeting we realized
there were many parallels within our aesthetics
and ways of thinking. The site became an outlet
for all the imagery we had collected, but
it also helped us move beyond being limited
to one discipline. From day one, we saw the blog
as an open window through which to share our
vision and encourage heightened perception of and
engagement with our surroundings. Crucially we
also wanted it to serve as a platform to showcase
work, blur boundaries and spread something
inspiring and worthwhile.

Patternity aims to merge the new with the timeless.
Although we're aware of what is happening in the
now, culturally it's more about the documentation
of pattern, from the mundane to the magnificent.
We love featuring new designers, inspired by their
skill, technique, ethos or innovation, but for
us their work could just as easily sit next to that
of someone long-forgotten or unknown. Susie Bubble
once described us as "cult pattern curators";
we are now exploring the possibilities of working
offline and making Patternity a more tactile
experience in the real world.'

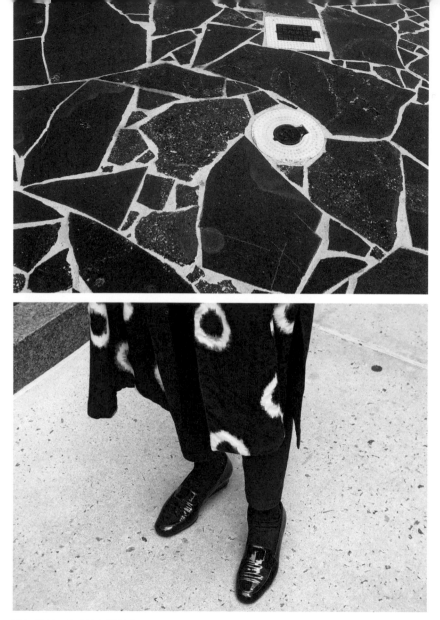

Top: Crazy paving patterns
Bottom: New York street style

Top: Puddle rainbow
Bottom: A crisscross of dusk shadows

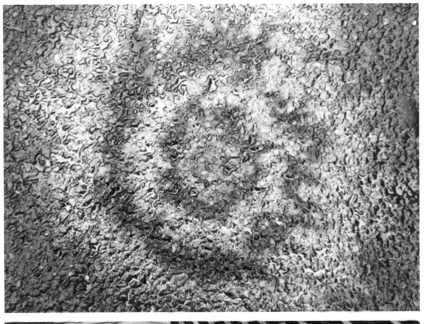

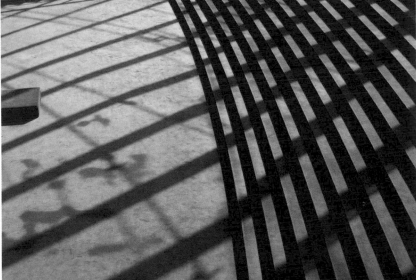

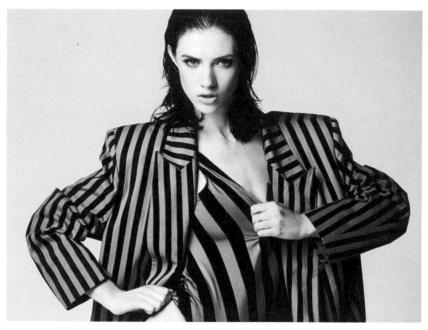

Miami Vice stripe

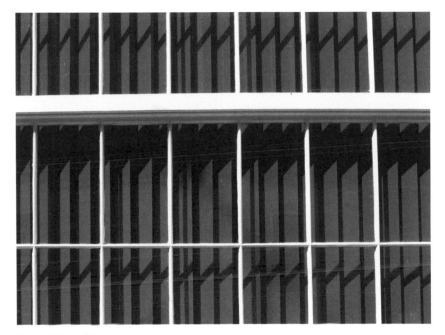

Red shutter grid

The Blonde Salad

Chiara Ferragni
theblondesalad.com

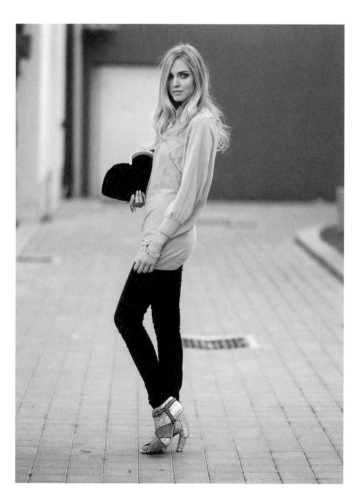

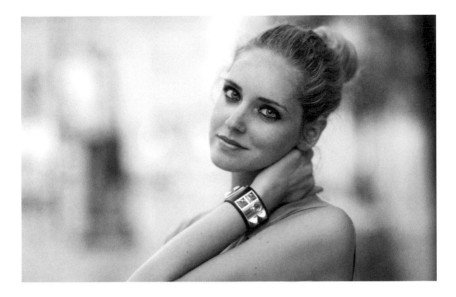

The Blonde Salad, Chiara Ferragni's personal journal of style, fashion and travel, has offered an all-encompassing glimpse into her glamorous and international life since 2009. It features behind-the-lens posts on location and interviews with designers and industry figures, including Tory Burch and Taylor Tomasi Hill, alongside her personal style inspirations. A law student at Bocconi University, the Milan-based blogger draws inspiration from the sartorial differences of varying cultures, looking to 'travel pictures and foreign blogs, which help open the mind to something new'. Charismatic and enthusiastic, her daily musings on fashion constitute a compelling blog which has seen her win both Bloglovin's Newcomer of the Year Award and the Blogger Business of the Year Award. Ferragni has designed capsule collections for labels such as Yamamay and the Werelse for Mango Touch project, while also contributing to the weekly publication *A Magazine*. She launched her own shoe line in 2010, further testament to the wide-ranging appeal of The Blonde Salad.

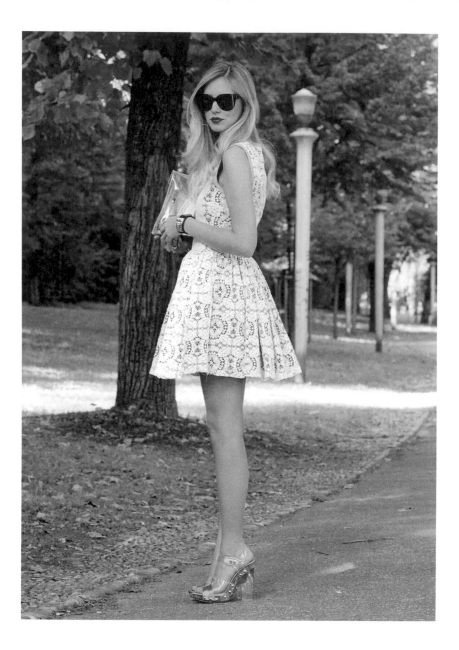

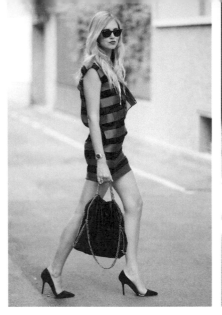
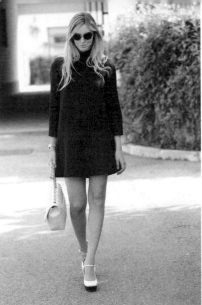

Chiara Ferragni

'Before beginning The Blonde Salad, I used to
share my outfit pics on Flickr, but then I realized
that I needed a more personal and unique space.
The blog is now my work and I feel very lucky
because I'm doing a lot of things connected to
it. The few hours I spend blogging are the best
of my day. I only cover things that I appreciate
because for me it is important to have a clear
relationship with my followers.

I don't have a specific style when it comes
to blogging because my taste is always evolving
and dependent on my mood. As an Italian, since
my country has a rich artistic heritage,
I grew up with a strong attraction to all that
is beautiful. That being said, I like it when
fashion follows the changes in our society and
the mix of different cultures.'

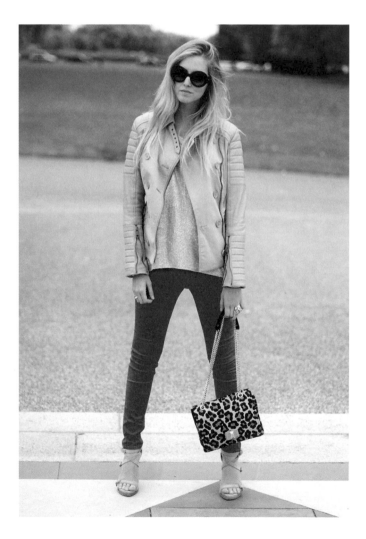

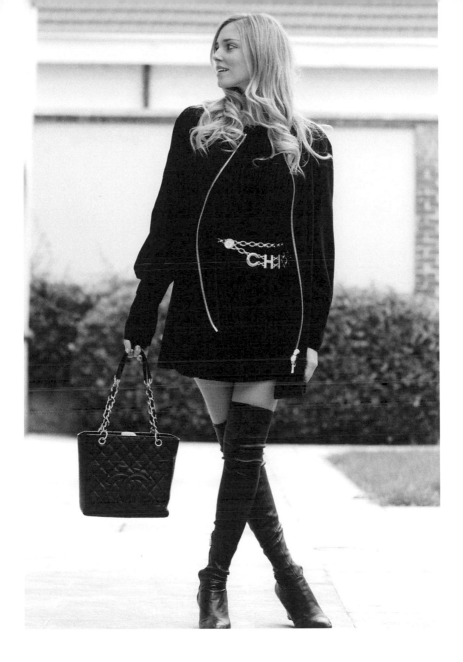

Stop It Right Now

Jayne Min

stopitrightnow.blogspot.com

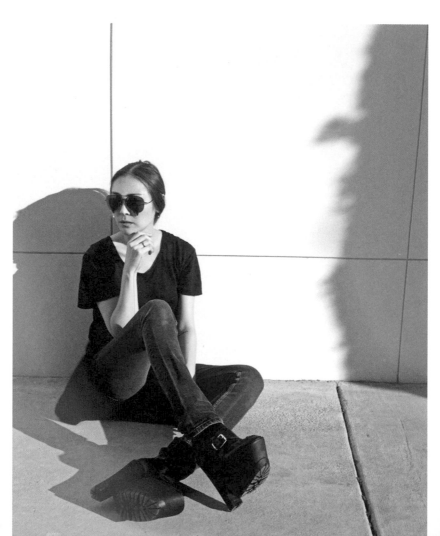

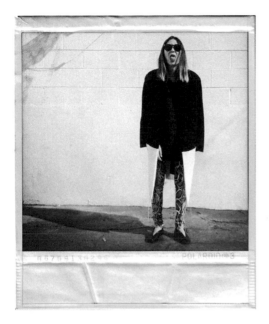

With her fresh combination of fashion-forward style obsession,
a love of skateboarding and her sense of tough, punked out
chic, Los Angeles-based Jayne Min has rapidly become the poster
girl for streetwear blogging. Stop It Right Now, founded in
2009, has an international following of girls and guys who look
to Min for style inspiration and admire her upfront attitude.
Coming from a background in apparel design, when Min first
started Stop It Right Now she had little experience with online
publishing: 'I had no idea what I was doing', she admits. Though
the blog's concept was not initially clearly defined, the result
is something that feels organic and natural, an online journal
that communicates her passions to an ever-growing audience.
Not settling for simply being known as a blogger, Min has also
designed a number of items, including skateboard decks and
handbags, that have been heralded across the web.

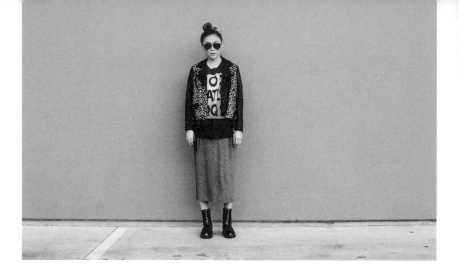

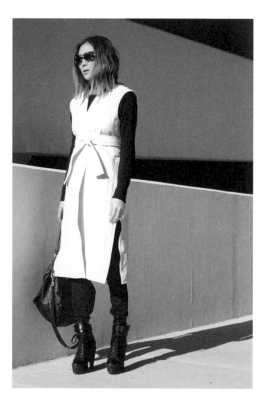

Jayne Min

'I approached Stop It Right Now as an online
journal to keep track of things I was into.
I really had no idea what I was getting myself
into. I think all blogs are fundamentally the
same in that bloggers generally post what
they like, and mine is no different, although
I have always tried not to post things that
have already circulated a bit. Original content
is always better.

One major thing that sets me apart may be my
age. I'm not a teenager so I think I attract
a certain kind of reader with a more discerning
eye. Something about the silhouette, textures
or colours of a piece or a designer's collection
has to really resonate with me in order for me
to feature it. I don't discriminate between styles
of designers or collections or seasons. I find
people in general inspiring and I find inspiration
in people's successes as well as their failures.

In the early days I was barely crawling out
of a totally analogue life and onto the Internet.
When I started observing other blogs, that's
when I knew I wanted to set myself apart. It
slowly transitioned into more original content
and a visual story that better represented me.
I also noticed my readership grew the more
of myself I shared. Stop It Right Now was never
intended to be a launching pad for a career
in fashion, so I have the rare luxury of really
not caring where it goes.'

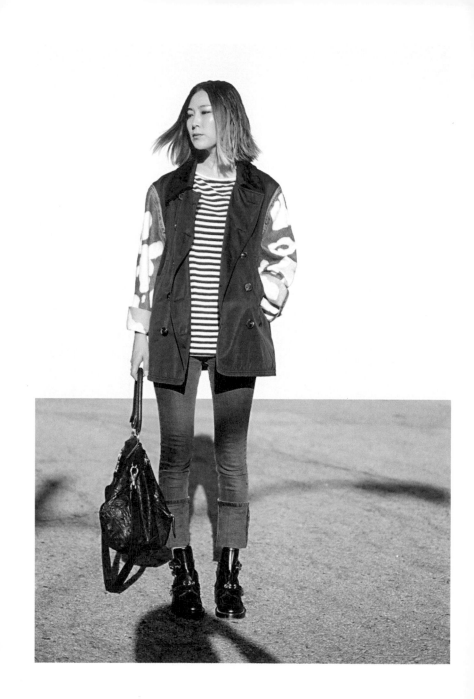

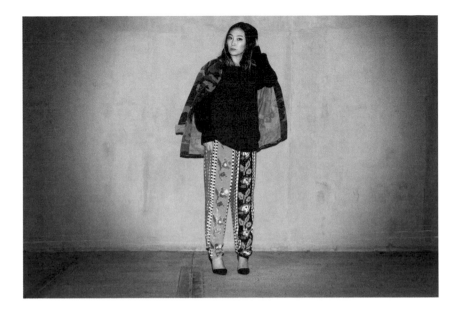

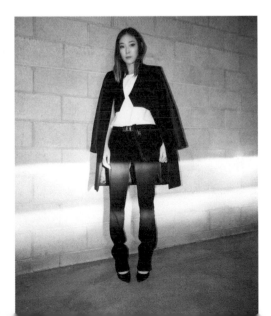

What Katie Wore

Joe Sinclair & Katie Mackay

whatkatiewore.co.uk

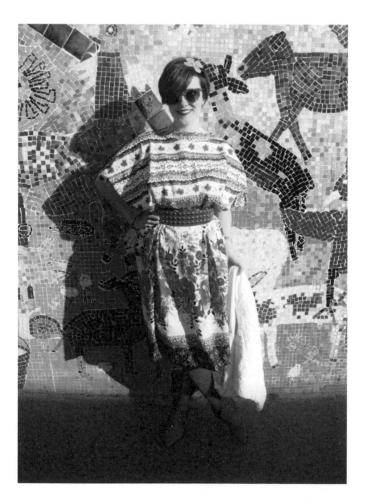

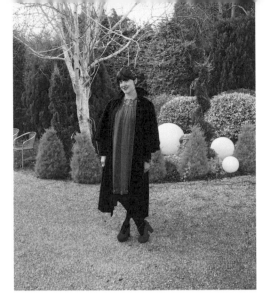

What Katie Wore, founded by Joe Sinclair and Katie Mackay
in 2009, had a simple premise: Mackay chose the outfit and
Sinclair photographed it and wrote an accompanying caption.
What started off as a challenge to wear an entirely different
outfit every day for twelve months subsequently turned into
a three-year project with thousands of dedicated readers.
To the London-based couple's surprise, their online endeavour
gained a cult following with over 5 million views from more
than 100 countries. Mackay's multifaceted, quirky and endlessly
varied style, described by her as 'playing dress-up at the end
of the rainbow', paired with Sinclair's spontaneous photography
and eloquent writing, made theirs a down-to-earth and genuine
contribution to the fashion blogging landscape. Completely
independent from trends or advertisers, it offered readers
a peek into its authors' everyday inspirations. Reflecting
on the blog's successful run, which ended in 2011, the couple
says: 'Every single bit of the What Katie Wore experience was
a highlight, but Anthony Burrill creating a bespoke print for
us to mark the end of the blog was something we'll never ever
forget.' Despite its ending, albeit on a high note, the online
legacy of the blog lives on.

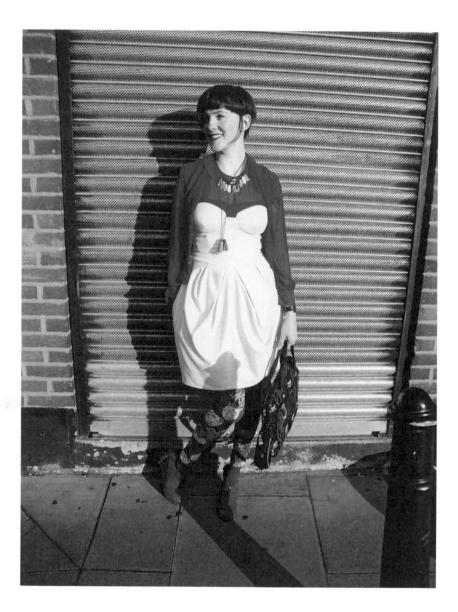

Katie Mackay

'I had been moaning that Joe never wrote me any love letters. Not being the love-letter-writing type, he decided to write a daily blog about me, promising to keep it up for as long as I could wear a different outfit every day. What Katie Wore was never a traditional fashion blog; we only ever featured pieces that I wanted to wear, rather than focusing on trends or designers. High-street, vintage, high-end, a hand-me-down from my mum, a gift from an independent designer starting out, a charity-shop find or something from Joe's wardrobe: all contributed to the eclectic style. What Katie Wore was always much more of a window into our lives than a fashion blog.

Blogging's prolific rise has certainly driven a broader rallying cry for the merits of personal style and so stretched the canvas on which eccentric, exciting and extraordinary style chameleons can be observed. It offers more perspectives on an industry that both thrives and depends on reinvention and constant spikes of inspiration.

What Katie Wore became as much a part of our daily lives as brushing our teeth. Even though we're not blogging any more, I'm still wearing something different (and brightly coloured) every day. I can't imagine that ever changing.'

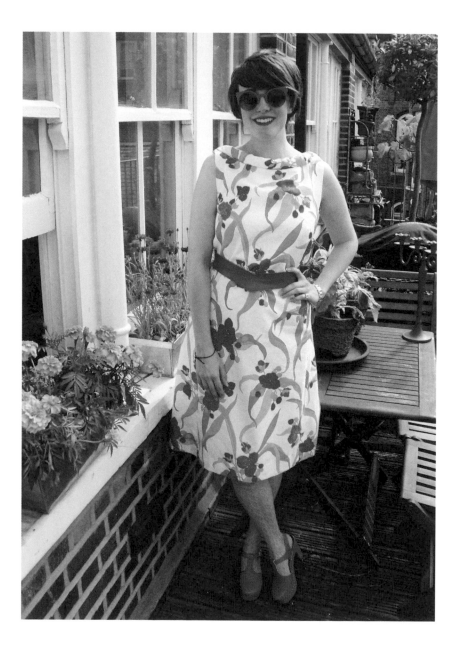

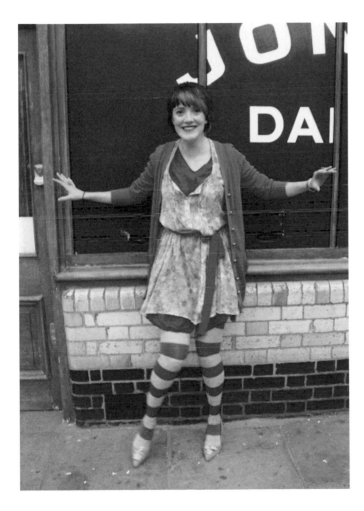

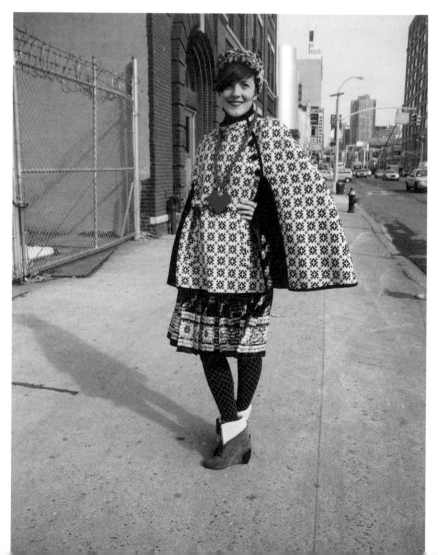

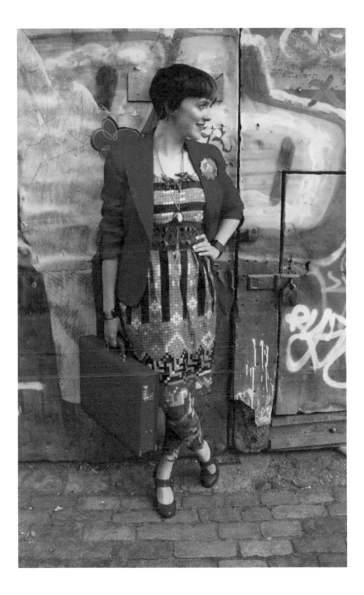

Cocorosa

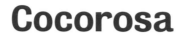

Chantal van der Meijden

mypreciousconfessions.blogspot.com

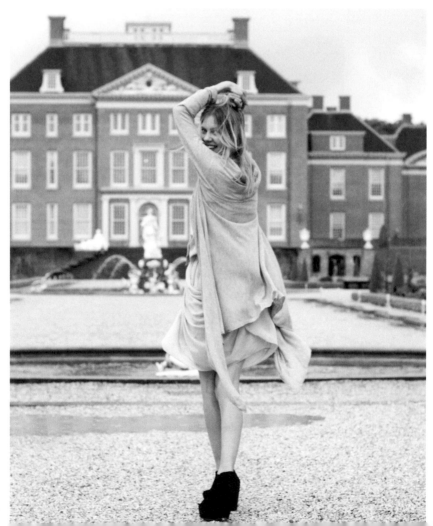

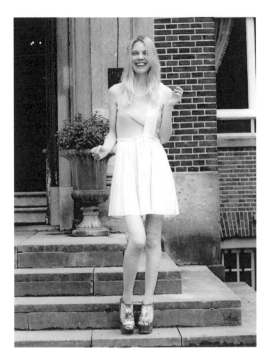

Following her work as a trend forecaster in New York and the realization that the styles she was seeing were often emerging from blogs, Chantal van der Meijden decided to start her own, Cocorosa, from the Netherlands in 2009. 'At the time the DIYs had a different mentality, trend- and consumer-wise, which I really liked. The blogs seemed like a perfect place to share creativity, inspire people to be creative and approach fashion in a different way', she explains. Centred on a combination of style posts and inspirational accessories, Van der Meijden sets out to show her readers how to style themselves, but also how to devise their own ideas. Her 'DIY Embellished Tights Tutorial' spread widely across the web and is testament to her distinctive point of view and the popularity of her styling. With a large base of readers coming to the site for its unique sense of colour and materials, Van der Meijden now focuses solely on the blog, bringing a hands-on element to the fashion world.

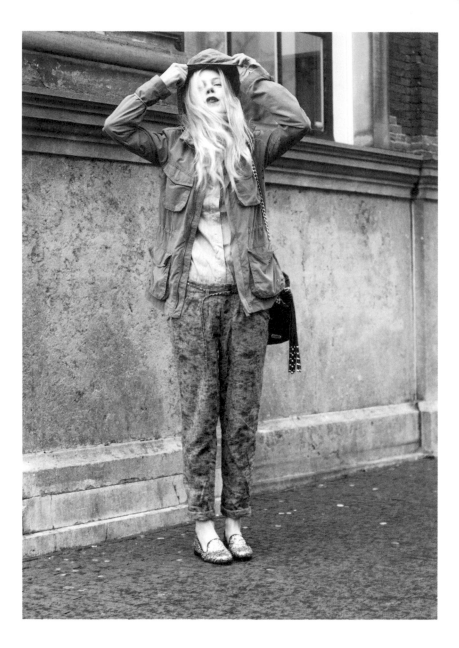

Chantal van der Meijden

'I really hate the feeling of being boxed in when it comes to everything in life, so for me it's important to always have that feeling of absolute freedom in whatever I do. I think people sense the freedom I feel when I do the things I love, so my blog is hopefully feelgood inspiration. When I was still working as a fashion trend forecaster my work used to be far more conceptual, so for me working on a commercial level is a challenge.

There are a lot of different blogs right now and all bring something different to the table. While some reflect the current fashion and consumer trends, others are true trendsetters and not only in fashion but in photography and editing. There are influencers, creators and more. I don't think I actually ever had a real concept for my blog except that I always followed my intuition, and that is still true. I always go with the flow and see where it takes me.'

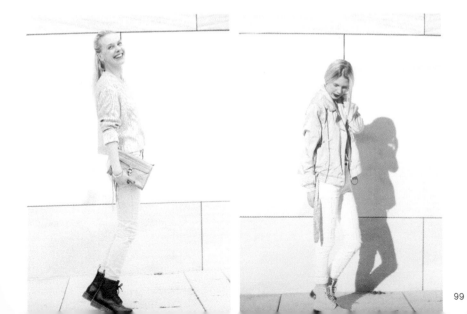

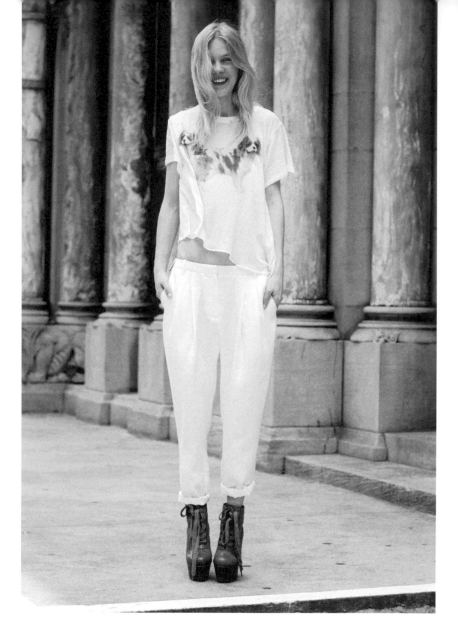

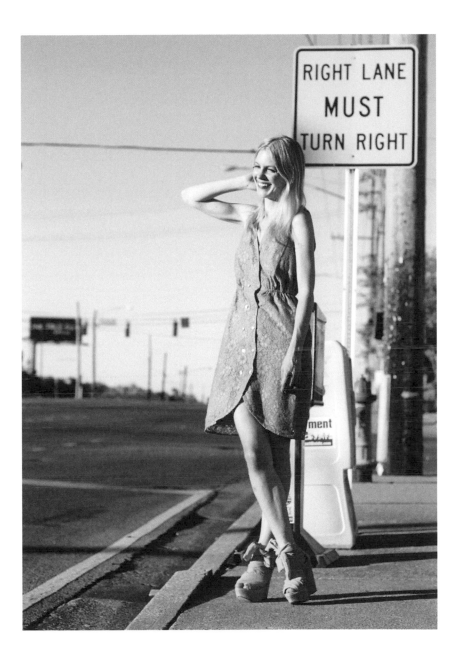

RIGHT LANE
MUST
TURN RIGHT

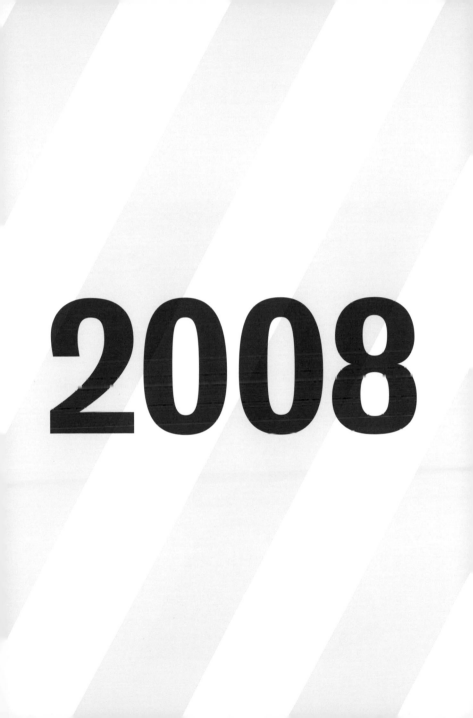

2008

Style Rookie

Tavi Gevinson

thestylerookie.com

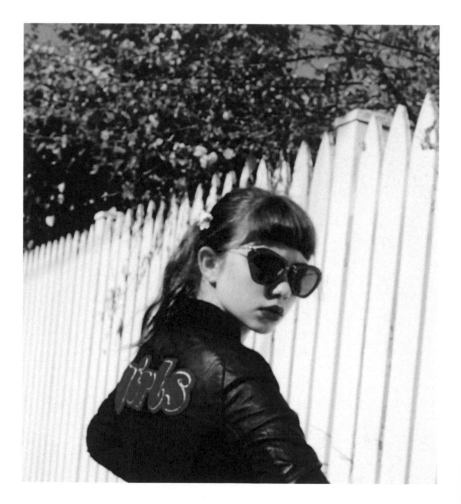

Tavi Gevinson has been blogging about fashion, fanzines and feminism from her family home in the suburbs of Chicago since March 2008. Initially gaining a following because of her young age – she founded Style Rookie at just 11 years old – Gevinson's sharp and alternative viewpoint and mix-and-match chic have endured, making her a sought-after fashion week attendee internationally. 'Mostly I am interested in American pop culture from the 1950s on, nostalgia and teen culture especially, so my style is full of the same kinds of knickknacks that would be on a messy teen's bedroom dresser', she explains. Gevinson is as intrigued by vintage and DIY garments as she is by Rei Kawakubo's Comme des Garçons, Meadham Kirchhoff and Proenza Schouler. Unlike most of her high-school peers, she has given TED Talks, is a contributing editor for *Garage Magazine* and is founder and editor-in-chief of *Rookie*, an online magazine for teenage girls launched in late 2011. 'With *Rookie* I want girls to feel like they are welcome to join the conversation', she says, 'to feel that they have an outlet, and that they can create their own outlet as well, and feel good about themselves.'

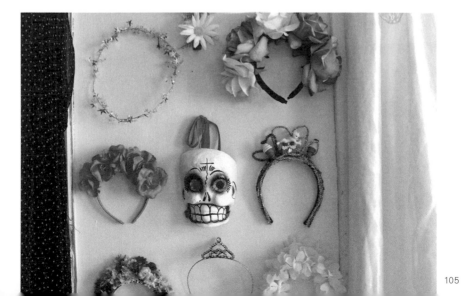

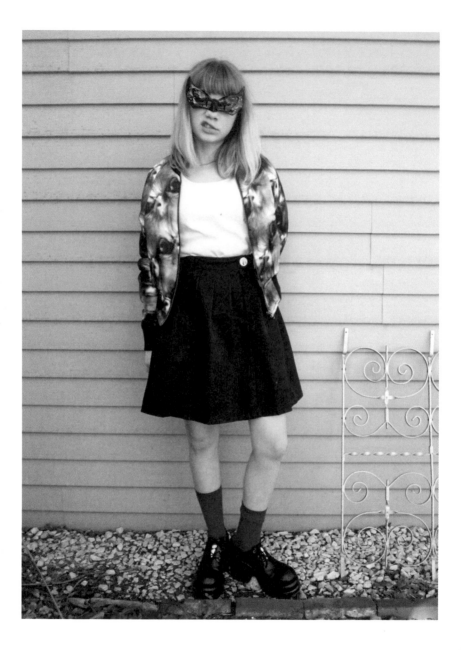

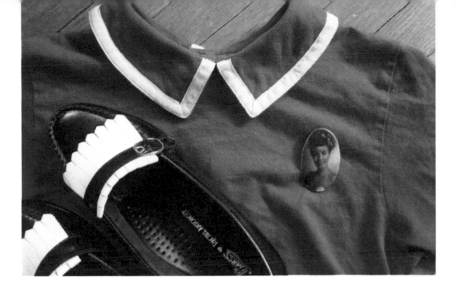

Tavi Gevinson

'I had been reading fashion blogs for some time
and wanted to find my style, and recording it all
online seemed like a convenient way to do so. The
older I've gotten, the less impressive my blog
should be, but people still seem to like it so
I guess there is something that makes it different.
Usually, though, my posts each have their own
aesthetics, so if it's a collection or something
that fits in with a bunch of other things I like at
the time, I'll tie them all together. On my own blog
I assume that the readers know me, but on Rookie
I don't quite take that tone. My blog is much more
train-of-thought and relaxed, just sort of figuring
out why I like certain things, and on Rookie I write
about those ideas once I feel I have figured it out
a bit more. I'm more nit-picky about the writing
that goes up on Rookie, since it's less about me
personally. It's much more edited than my own blog.
I just hope readers of Style Rookie enjoy it and
feel a little inspired or curious.'

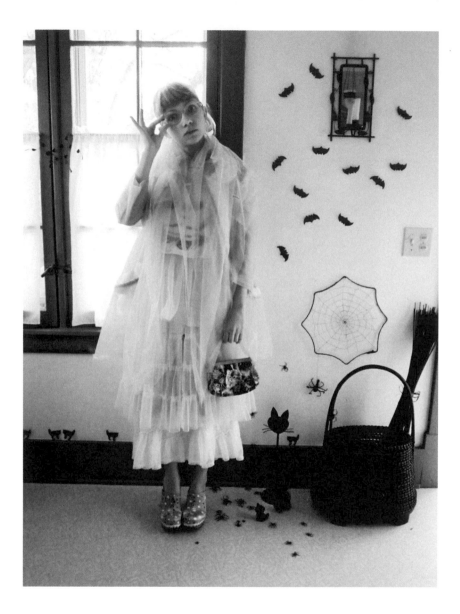

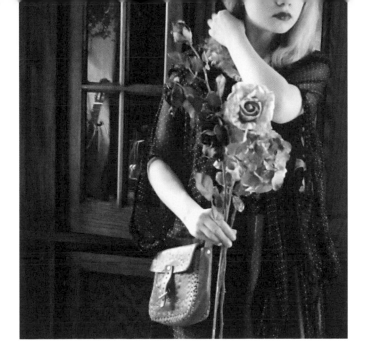

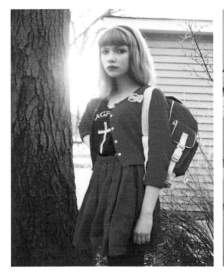

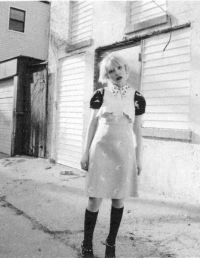

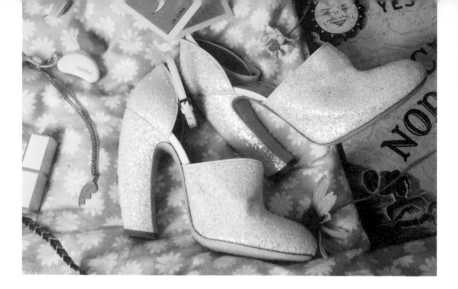

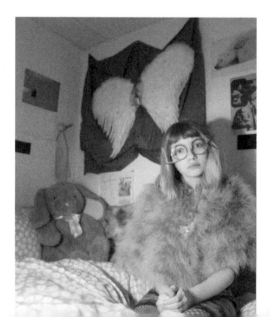

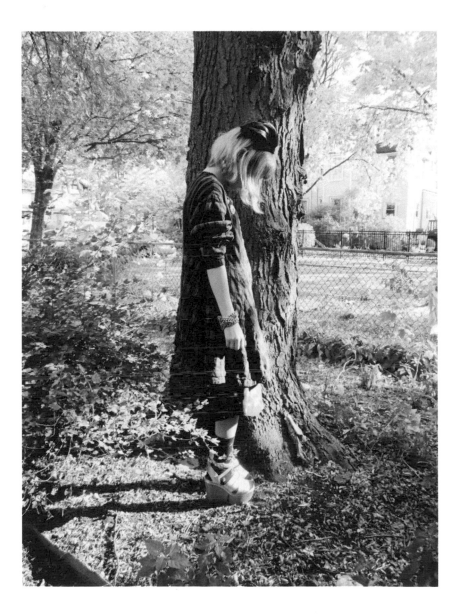

Advanced Style

Ari Seth Cohen

advancedstyle.blogspot.com

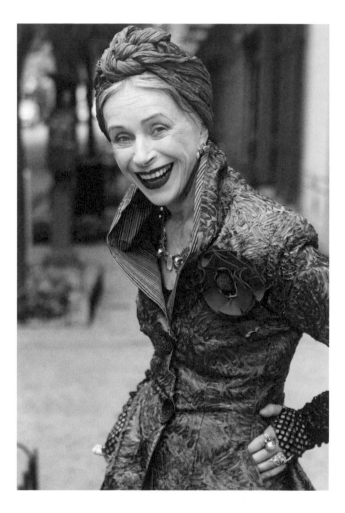

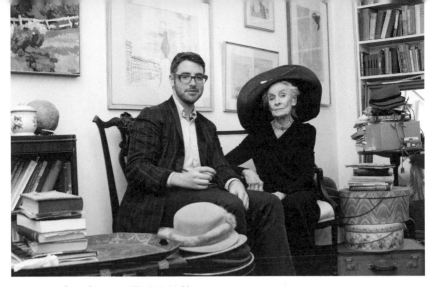

Above: Ari Seth Cohen and Mimi Weddell
Opposite: Beatrix Ost

Working as a freelance photographer and writer, in 2008 Ari Seth
Cohen started his blog dedicated to 'the sartorial splendor
of the silver-haired set'. Advanced Style focuses on an older
generation who maintain a passionate interest in the way
they dress, with Cohen capturing his chic and dapper subjects
mainly on the streets of New York, as well as internationally.
The timeless yet contemporary images are often accompanied
by eloquent descriptions from Cohen, who studied art history
at the University of Washington. He discusses the inspiration
he draws from the outfits he sees and his experiences of meeting
and photographing his models, but also how he is influenced
by the people he meets. Cohen has an authentic love for his
subjects and his excitement about meeting new, strikingly
dressed elders shines through in his blog. Advanced Style is
praised for its elegant aesthetic, while Cohen counts appearing
on *The Today Show* as one of the highlights of his blogging
career. He currently lectures on the subject of advanced style,
a book of images and interviews from the blog has been published
and a documentary film is in the works.

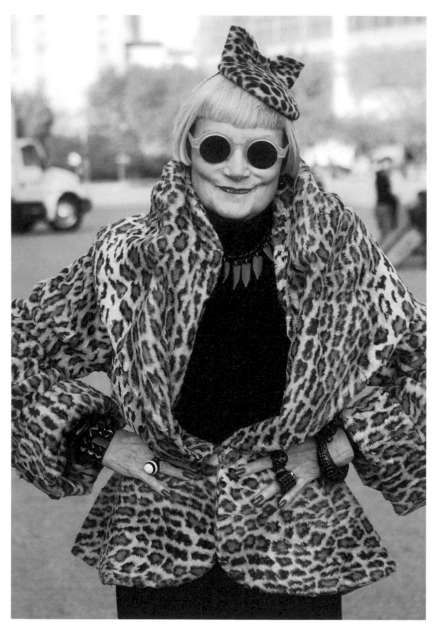

Joana Avillez

Ari Seth Cohen

'I feature people who follow their own trends –
people with great stories and unique personal
style, Cary Grant mixed with Anna Piaggi and
Quentin Crisp. I focus on men and women over 60,
a demographic often ignored by the fashion media.

I am inspired by other bloggers who look outside
of themselves for inspiration. I look at blogs that
present a unique perspective and a very personal
point of view. The platform allows a diverse range
of voices to be heard and bloggers can freely
express fresh ideas and opinions without having
to please consumers and advertisers. The trick
is to stay true to your vision. I have always had
the same goals but over the past few years
I have had more time to commit to Advanced Style.
I have developed a network of subjects and can
concentrate more fully on the stories behind their
personal styles. My blog has developed beyond
style – it is about lifestyle.'

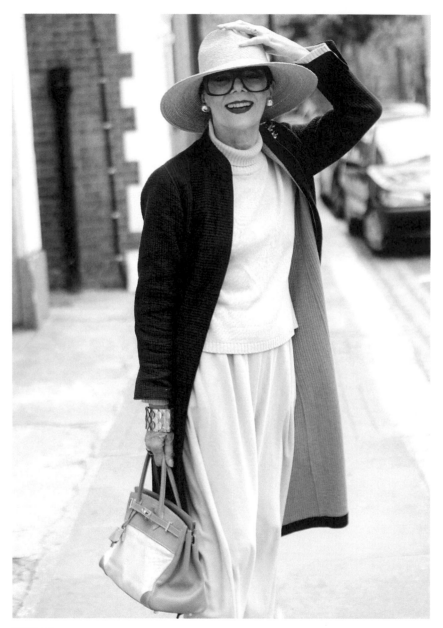

Gitte Lee

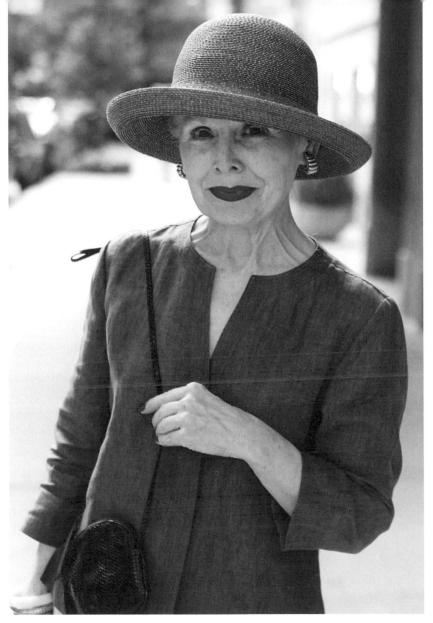

Advanced Style on Madison Avenue

The Dandy Project

Izzy Tuason
thedandyproject.com

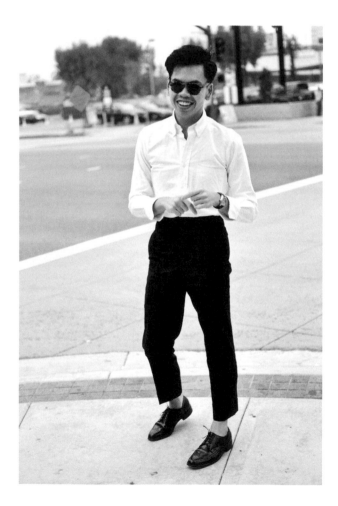

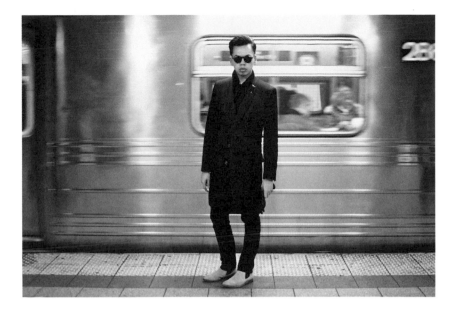

Izzy Tuason's The Dandy Project is a refreshing alternative
to the majority of menswear blogs, featuring a combination
of self-style posts, profiles on high-end designers and emerging
names, and guides on how to create DIY garments alongside
musings on must-have pieces and opinions on the industry itself.
Pattern, colour, texture and clean, minimal styling all coincide
in Tuason's take on men's fashion in New York. The site aims
to help its readers to be experimental while retaining a sense
of masculinity. At the core of The Dandy Project is an evolving
interest in craftsmanship and detail. Accessories, often
overlooked by menswear blogs, are a distinct interest of Tuason's
and he regularly features jewellery designers alongside bag-
and shoemakers. While working as a marketing professional,
which included freelance writing and styling for various
print and online publications, Tuason started the blog after
seeing the coverage a friend of his was rapidly garnering
with her simple site. Now an established blogger, he travels
internationally with his site and has been selected to
collaborate with various brands and other blogs.

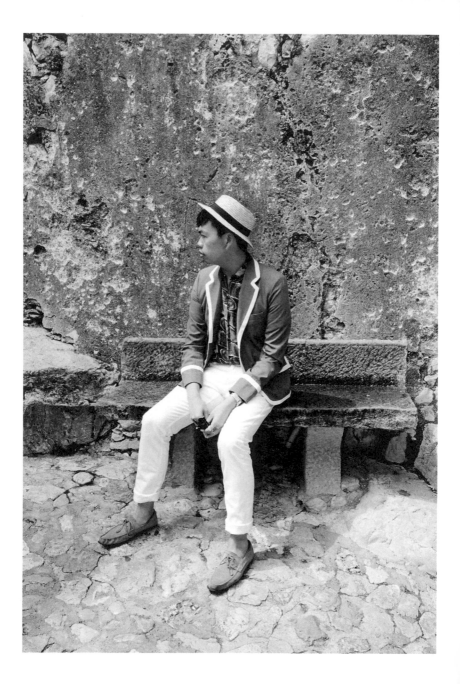

Izzy Tuason

'I was fascinated at how a medium as easy
and personal as blogging could potentially be
a megaphone for anybody with something worthwhile
to say. I slowly inched my way into the blogosphere,
first uploading outfit photos on The Fashion Spot's
"What are you wearing today?" thread, and in 2008
I started The Dandy Project. It took a few months
for me to be comfortable enough to stop cutting
my head off in photos of myself and a few more
months to think about doing DIY posts. If I see
something that makes my eyes widen, my heart skip
a beat or makes me smile, I have to blog about it.
I like designers who embrace creativity and
freedom in their work, who bring something new
to our collective creative consciousness. I don't
like rules. I appreciate good tailoring and will
always be more dressed up than the average guy
at the office. I gravitate towards darkness, believe
in quality over quantity, and never take fashion
too seriously.

The best blogs, despite being kept afloat
by sponsors, never lose their personal voice.
I love how fashion blogging has helped champion
diversity in dressing. The ease with which one
can start blogging and the potential to reach
so many people has helped minorities and people
with unusual tastes find a niche. I was a bow-
tie fanatic at the inception of the blog,
so I thought it befitting to name that little
project of mine "dandy". I've since grown out
of traditional manifestations of dandyism, but
kept the name, even though I interpret it in
a looser, more modern way.'

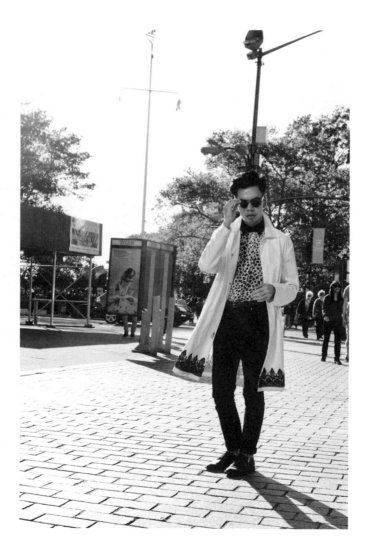

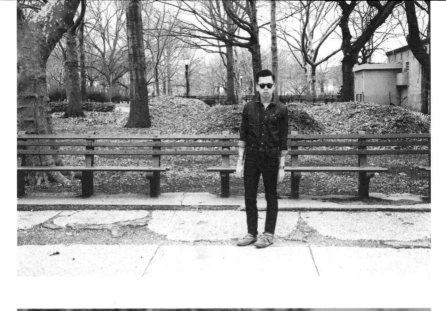

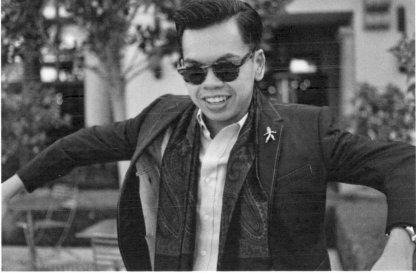

Jak & Jil

Tommy Ton
jakandjil.com

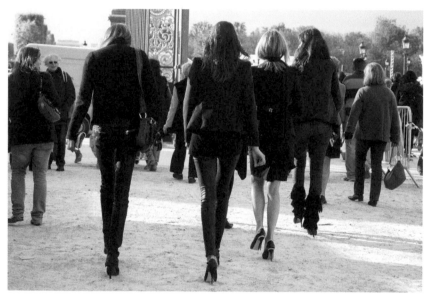

Paris

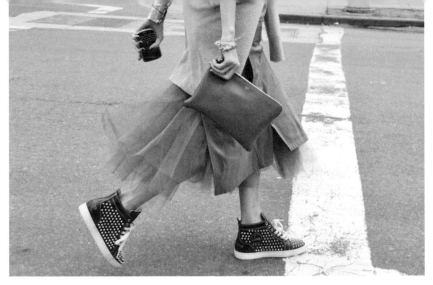

New York

Based in Ontario, Canada, but travelling to fashion month
proceedings around the globe, Tommy Ton of Jak & Jil has become
one of the most revered style bloggers around. His upfront,
colourful and intelligent images, often with a distinct sense
of knowing humour, have captured the great and the good from
the world of fashion. Voyeuristically catching editors,
designers, models and attendees as they walk or stand waiting
for shows, Ton highlights clothes and their textures and colours
in a way that is uniquely his own. To differentiate his blog
from others, Ton chooses to focus on details, whether shoes,
patterns or a clash of materials. After he started the online
image gallery back in 2008, the site rapidly led to a number
of high-profile jobs. Ton has gone on to shoot for many magazines
and websites, has earned himself positions at both Style.com and
GQ.com and has become one of the most sought-after attendees
at industry events internationally.

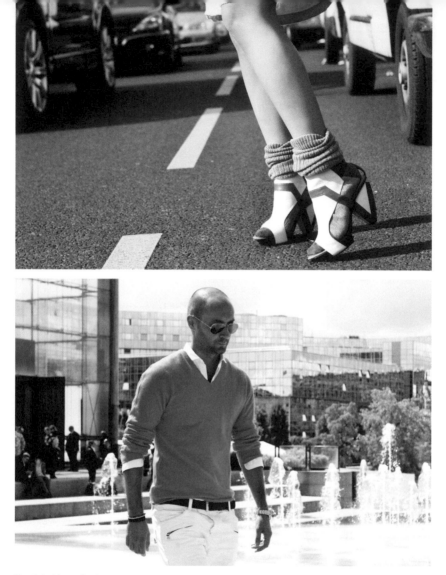

Top & bottom: Paris

Tommy Ton

'The blog came about organically after I realized I had too many photos from my travels in fashion month. It has given me more opportunities to work in the industry and if anything has challenged me to work harder and have more of an open mind about fashion and the Internet. The blog certainly motivates me to keep working. Everybody does different things with blogging, but it's the people who have a distinct point of view that stand out. I'm just putting out there what I find visually stimulating and hope it is of interest to others. It has to be distinctive and very much from a personal point of view that is relatable and accessible. I can appreciate avant-garde design, but I really value someone who thinks very hard about what people want and need.

I love looking at other people's blogs every day. They inspire me to think outside the box, to focus more on being myself and to refine my narrative. Blogging has democratized fashion in so many ways. It's turned fashion into an open forum in which anyone can voice their opinion and the sense of immediacy it has brought has certainly changed the pace of the industry.'

London

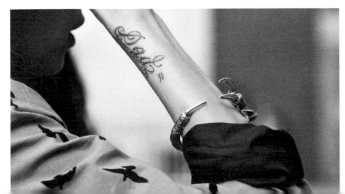

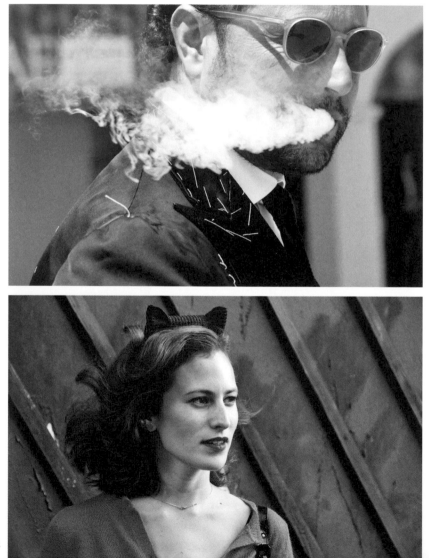

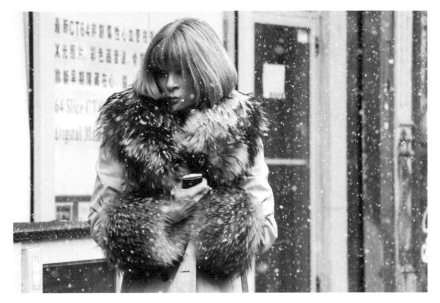

Above: New York
Overleaf: Milan

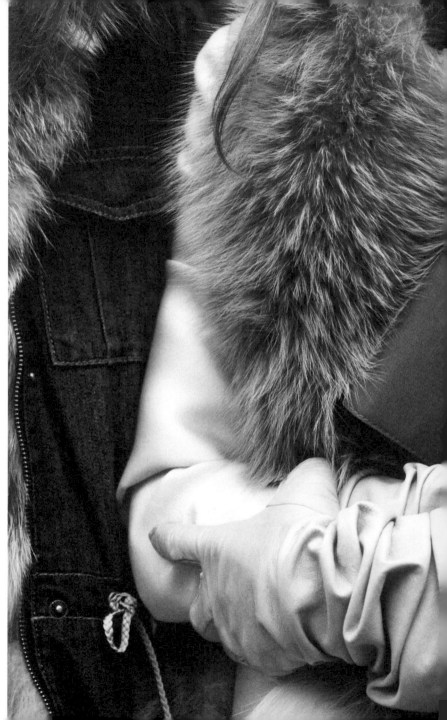

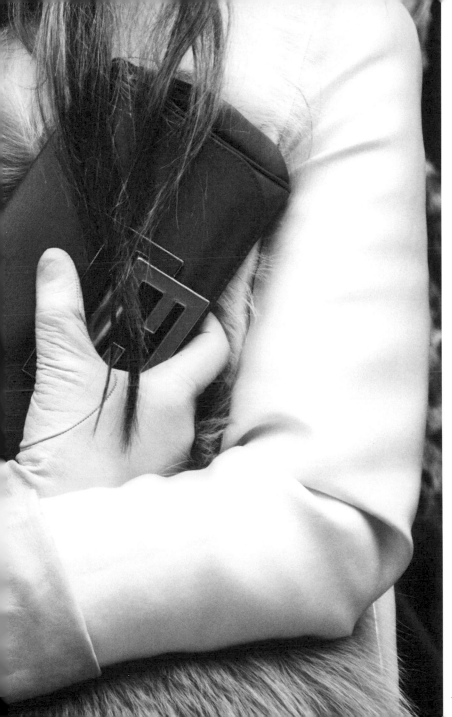

Lulu and Your Mom

Lulu Chang

luluandyourmom.blogspot.com

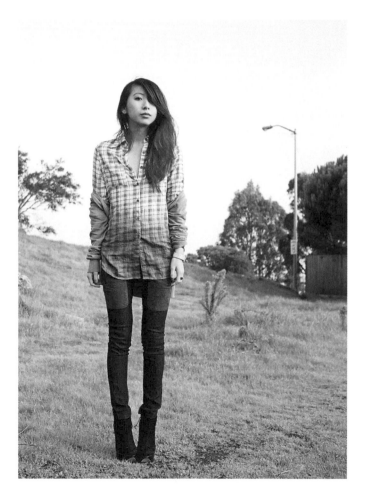

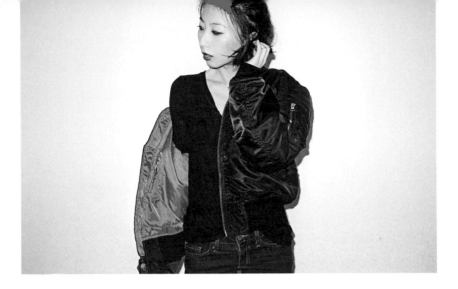

With her striking look, upfront attitude and carefully selected style choices that combine high-end fashion with streetwear, Lulu Chang has been termed the 'It Girl' of the San Francisco fashion scene with her blog Lulu and Your Mom, founded in 2008. Chang has a distinctive take on a classic feminine look with elements of androgyny mixed in. Her blog is an online style diary covering her experimentation with different clothes, her love of discovery and her strong opinions. While she does promote brands, designers and key pieces, shopping is not the main subject of the blog. Chang looks to create a 'global brand', as she herself describes it, a place where readers can come for inspiration and subsequently source the items she curates themselves. Also working as a designer, she has an innate sense of how to put outfits together with a constant nod towards the empowering and the chic. The site has led to Chang co-authoring *The Fashion Coloring Book* and co-founding the womenswear label The Fashion Club.

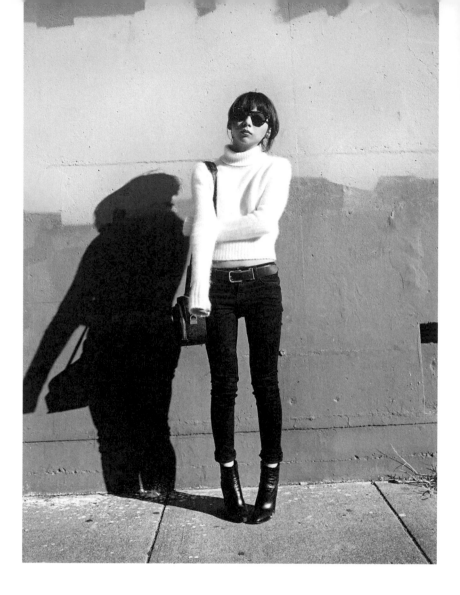

Lulu Chang

'I've been a follower of fashion on the web for quite some time. One day my friend was looking over my shoulder at a blog I was reading and told me, "You could do that. I think people would really like you."

I don't like to make shopping the focus of my blog. I believe the product, brand or designer I feature has to align with my aesthetic but, even more importantly, it has to promote something new. I'm really into an exchange of ideas. As a designer, I feel that this is just as important as selling your latest handbag. It's necessary to put things in context; it's about the story. It's about beauty and love. In general I find people inspiring and blogging brings a personal element to making and sharing ideas. If you lose your voice, you lose your content.'

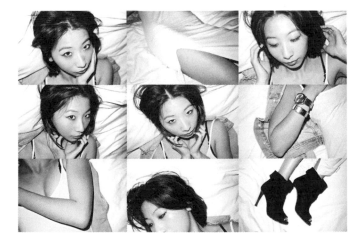

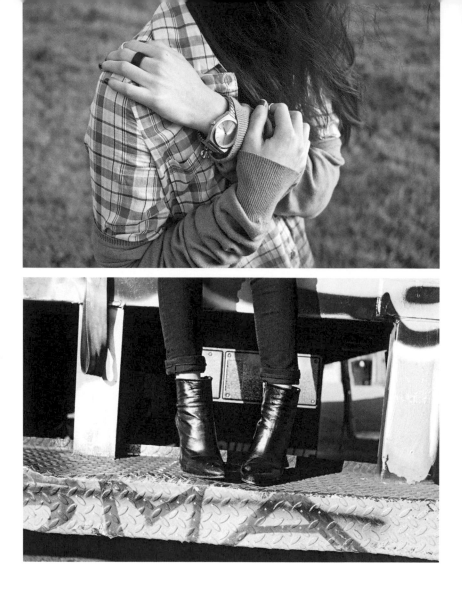

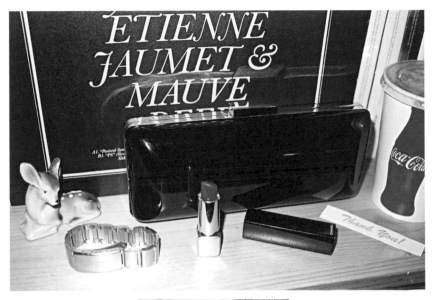

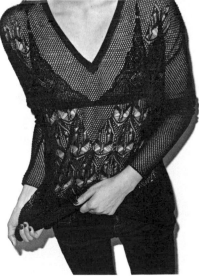

Hapsical

Peter Henderson

hapsical.blogspot.co.uk

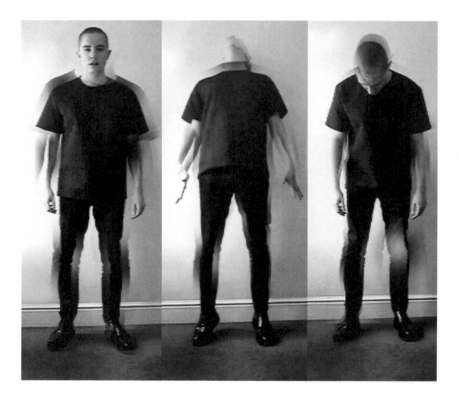

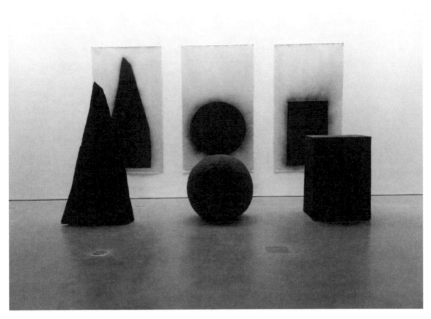

David Nash exhibition, Yorkshire Sculpture Park

Obsessed with a dark, modernist take on menswear, London-based blogger Peter Henderson founded Hapsical in 2008 as a way for the then-student to cover his love of a refined, forward-thinking code of dress. Rather than featuring a host of designers or following current trends, Henderson tends to look to a handful of names – Raf Simons, Yves Saint Laurent, Lanvin, Maison Martin Margiela and Rick Owens – for inspiration. His colour of choice is black and in his posts he creates an aesthetic with industrial, futurist and minimalist references. Hapsical also pulls in information on artists and musicians that fit this focused and defined style. It has garnered some high-profile fans, notably Raf Simons himself, who read one of Henderson's posts and subsequently invited him to be part of the Avant/Garde Diaries: Transmission 1 culture festival held in Berlin in 2011. Now also working as a fashion writer for menswear site Mr Porter, at the age of just 21, Henderson has already staked his claim on the fashion world.

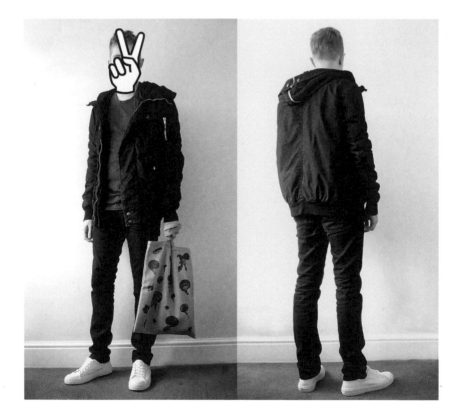

Peter Henderson

'I was passionate about fashion and a bit
of a closet computer nerd, so I thought, "Maybe
I can do this blogging thing too." I only feature
things I am genuinely interested in; life's too
short to create posts to please PRs or advertisers.
I have that luxury because I don't make any money
from Hapsical: I don't owe anybody coverage.
I like modernism, minimalism and clean lines set
against elements of style associated with youth
subcultures, from skinheads to skaters.

To start with, I didn't have much of a vision: lots
of fashion news, pictures of products and magazine
editorials. I really cringe when I look back at
my early posts, especially because I used to write
as "we" to make it sound more professional - as
if there was a Hapsical team! As countless other
fashion blogs came into existence doing the same,
I realized there's no point in trying to play
the successful commercial blogs at their own
game. These days I do a mixture of outfit posts,
travel photos and lengthy written posts
exploring particular designers or the workings
of the fashion industry in depth, mixed in with
a "curated" selection of things I find inspiring,
from fashion, architecture and art to design.

My blog helped me to get my current job as
well as the internships I did beforehand. It's
one thing to say on your CV that you love fashion
and can write, but if you have a body of work
online proving the point, it can make all the
difference. Blogs have definitely shaken up
the fashion establishment, which I think is
mostly a good thing.'

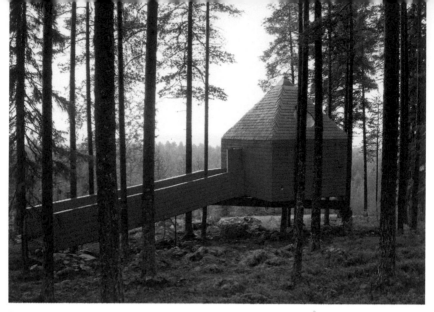

The Treehotel, Sweden

Prada Resort 2012

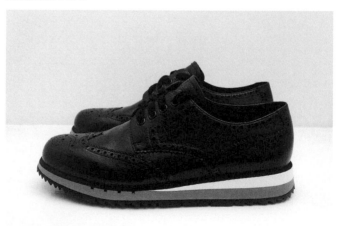

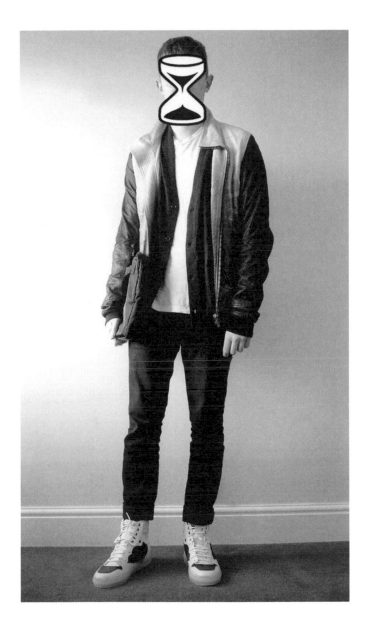

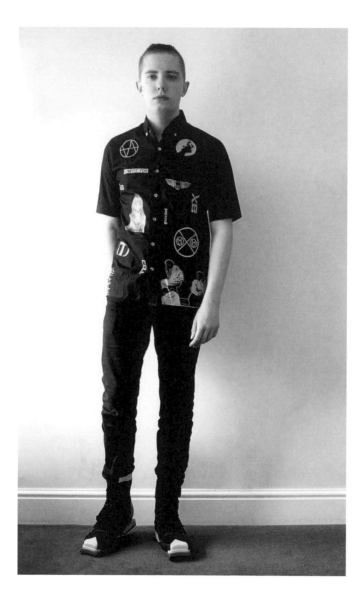

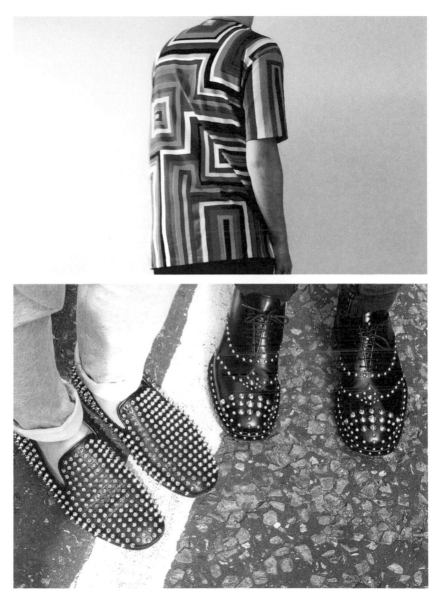

Bottom: L to R: Tommy Ton in Christian Louboutin shoes,
Peter Henderson in Prada shoes

Karla's Closet

Karla Deras

karlascloset.com

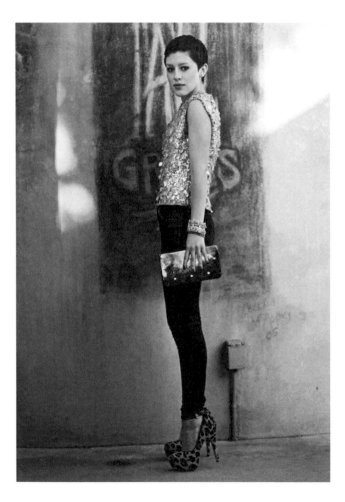

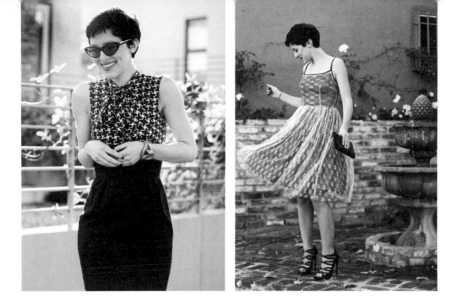

After earning a degree in apparel manufacturing from the
Fashion Institute of Design and Merchandising, Los Angeles,
and a brief stint in the all-American girl-pop group Slumber
Party Girls, Karla Deras started Karla's Closet in 2008. The
blog focuses on her own personal style, but it features posts
on high-end pieces and her favourite designers (including
Versace, Prada, Louboutin and Balenciaga) alongside images
of customized or restyled vintage finds. Inspired to start her
own blog after avidly reading many others, Deras is now an
established part of the professional blogging community. She
has her own army of readers eager to find inspiration in her
unique, chic and urban way of dressing. Coming from a personal
angle, using the blog as a way of communicating her love of the
things she comes across or obsesses over, her posts capture
her excitement and passion for her outfits. 'I was a big reader
of blogs like The Sartorialist and Style Bubble and got inspired
to start my own. I wanted an outlet to talk about fashion,
since none of my friends were into it', she says. Since she
started to blog, Deras's profile has grown rapidly, giving her
the opportunity to work with a variety of brands and designers,
including Coach and Macy's.

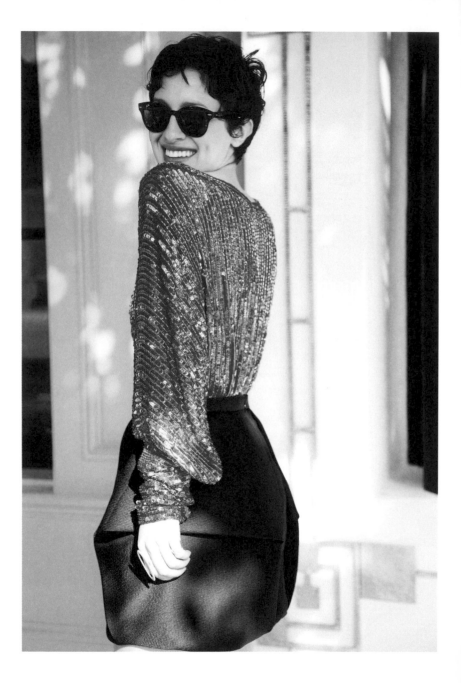

Karla Deras

'I have to love something in order to wear
it on my blog – whether it's an Elizabeth and
James jumpsuit or a 1950s swing skirt. Everything
I cover is an extension of me in some way. I'd say
my aesthetic is very experimental yet classic.
I know what I feel good in, but I like to take
risks. I love mixing my mood and feelings with
colours, themes and shapes.

As soon as I graduated, I started blogging
full-time. I didn't really have any idea of what
I wanted to do with my blog at first but I always
knew I wanted to post quality content. Every
project I work on has something to do with my blog
and I am definitely inspired by other blogs, from
interior design to beauty. Sometimes I'm inspired
by the way a photograph is captured and at other
times it can be something as simple as wanting
to try a new mascara that I read about. I think
influential blogs are a great platform for brands
because they allow them to convey their brand
messages and engage with the blog's audience.'

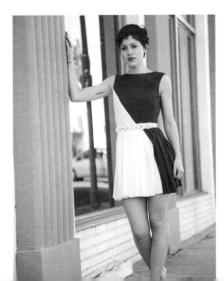
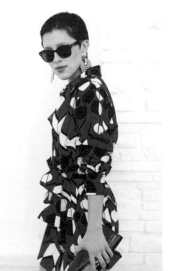

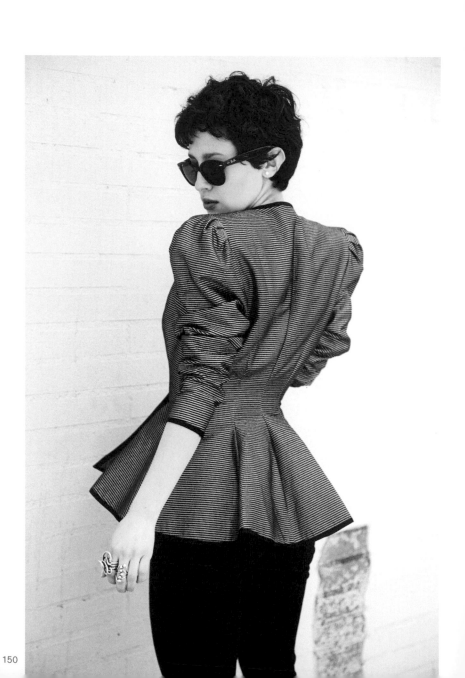

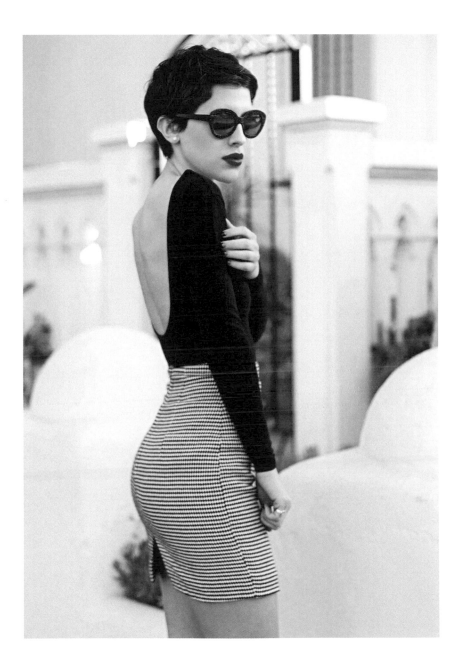

Luxirare

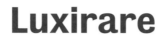

Ji Kim

luxirare.com

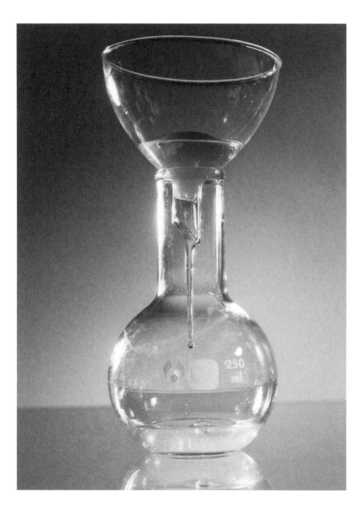

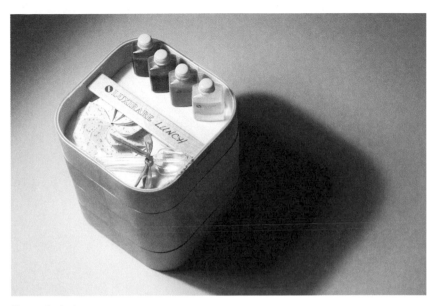

Above: Bento box
Opposite: Egg yolk and egg white separation for oyster consommé

A mix of food, recipes, ideas, clothes and inspiration, Ji Kim's
Luxirare is the go-to blog for a little bit of New York chic.
Founded in 2008, the site elegantly profiles everything that its
author deems interesting or relevant to her lifestyle. Image-
heavy posts of beautiful people and items are aligned with
Kim's outspoken opinions on the fashion world and her style
values. Kim's aesthetic is made up of glamorous, empowered
classic and street styles all mixed together. With an ardent
following of everyday readers, industry professionals and
other serious bloggers, Kim has made her mark and is continuing
to do so with features on her culinary and stylistic ideas in
books and magazines and on websites. Alongside the main blog,
Luxirare also features a journal with more spontaneous posts
and an e-shop containing pieces designed by Kim herself
as well as those by other brands and designers.

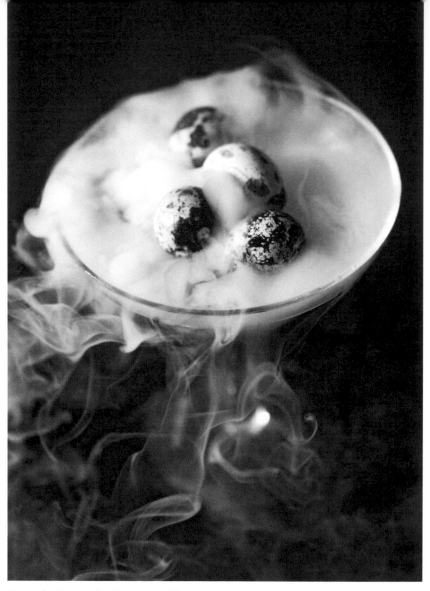

Above: Quail eggs for ikura handroll pieces
Overleaf: Truffle honey

Ji Kim

'In the beginning I didn't see a fashion blog that integrated the process and presentation of food, so that was something that I wanted to contribute through mine. I knew, with so many hardworking, talented fashion bloggers out there, it would be very difficult and challenging to offer anything better, but I thought it would be a nice idea to start with. I thought there had to be other people out there who understood that the two were not so different, at least in their consumption and execution style.

On the fashion side of things, I tend to feature a good deal of Alaïa, Helmut Lang, Raf Simons and Gianni Versace's older designs. It's important to me that a designer has a strong world to communicate and these designers are people who have defined their worlds very clearly.

I believe it's important to share images or designs that have not circulated around the other major blogs, to offer something to my readers that they might have not seen before. From the start, my presentation style on the website has been very minimal. I don't tend to add any frivolous elements, at least when it comes to photography or storytelling. Items and food are generally presented as directly as possible, usually on a white background. In the beginning I did feel as though maybe this style was not enough, that it could be a little more editorial or lavish, but right now I feel very comfortable with it. I really love reading fashion blogs; they provide a peek into a world in which you may never live.'

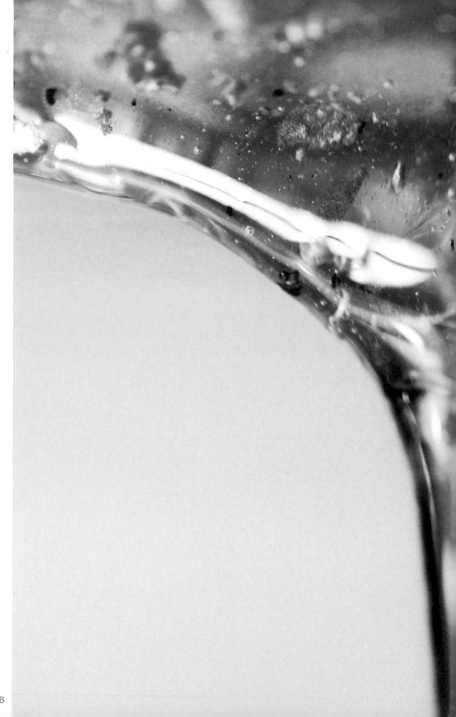

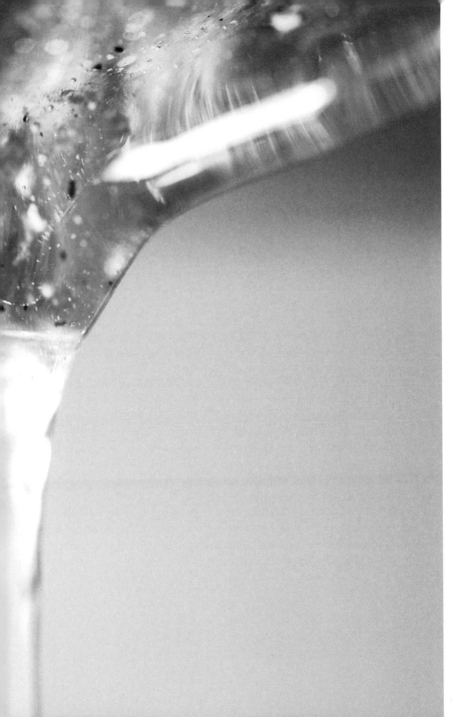

Dapper Kid

Syed Ahsan Abbas

dapperkid.blogspot.co.uk

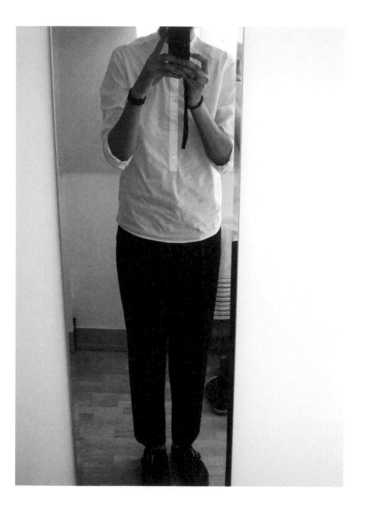

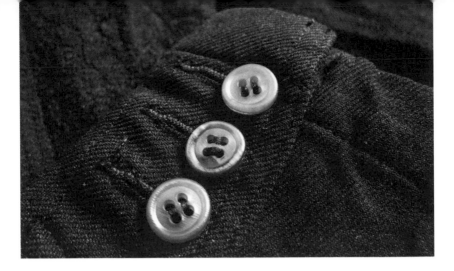

Providing an insight into his intellectualized relationship with fashion and design, London-based art history student Syed Ahsan Abbas's Dapper Kid is known for its intriguing writing and the author's classic and minimalist style values. Covering mainly menswear, the site is an evaluation of the design landscape as he sees it, with discussions of his own experiences, emotions and relationships with items. He has a concise grasp of the values he is looking for and the references within a collection while being able to describe the collaboration between these elements effectively and poetically. His focus is often on a more unique sense of style - something with innovative contrasting textures, embellishment and a sense of humour, or a more restrained, simple and dark silhouette. Abbas also shows editorial layouts and campaigns that have interested or inspired him, again looking for innovation combined with an underlying depth from both photographer and stylist. Not purely restricted to fashion, Dapper Kid interposes its posts with features on artists, illustrators and other creatives.

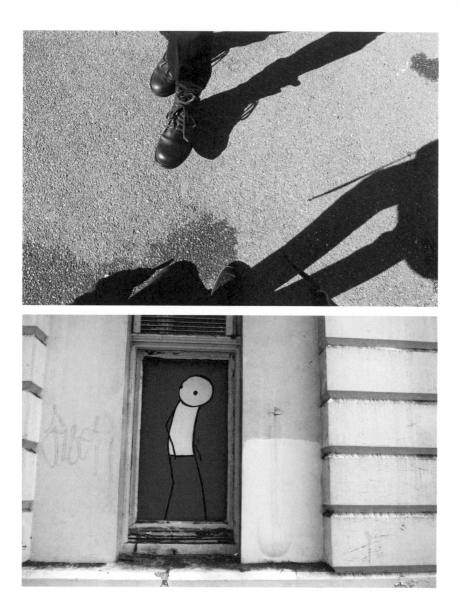

Syed Ahsan Abbas

'The blog was and is a mix of designers, collections, garments, editorials, images, videos, ideas and issues that interest me. I use it as a forum in which to explore ideas around fashion design and the fashion system. I am attracted to designers who have a strong personal aesthetic and a design philosophy and ethos that I identify with. I return to the same few designers again and again simply because they are the ones whose work and style I most enjoy and relate to. My blog is and always has been personal: it will always be about the designers who are important to me, rather than whoever is popular at the time.

With my blog I sometimes try to examine fashion from a physical perspective, using the experience of the wearer, because the ultimate purpose of the garment is to be worn. Discussing an image and discussing a physical garment are two very different things, but I try to do both because I am interested in all aspects of fashion and dress. Barthes argued that fashion can never truly be represented through text, but it is one of the few media we have, and perhaps the most expressive one.

I think fashion blogging adds a much-needed sense of approachability to the industry. Fashion can be notoriously scary and confusing for the outsider, so for someone to be able to find a place where it is presented and discussed in an accessible manner is vital.'

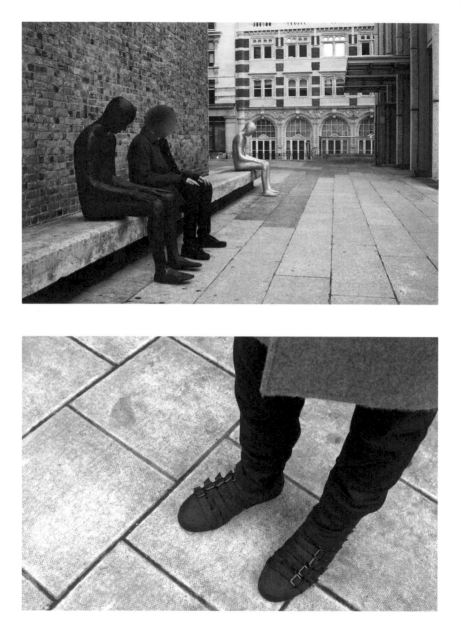

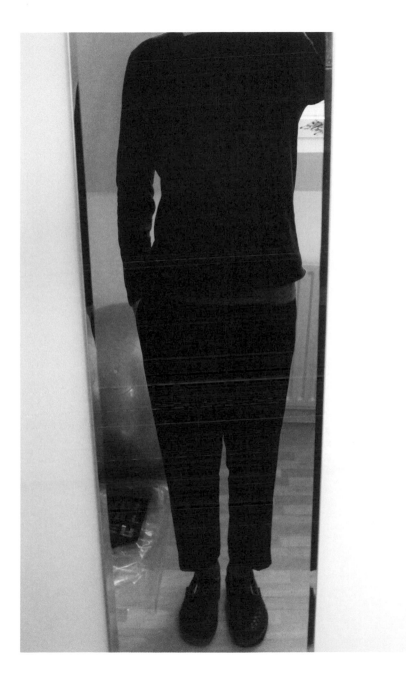

Vanessa Jackman

Vanessa Jackman

vanessajackman.blogspot.co.uk

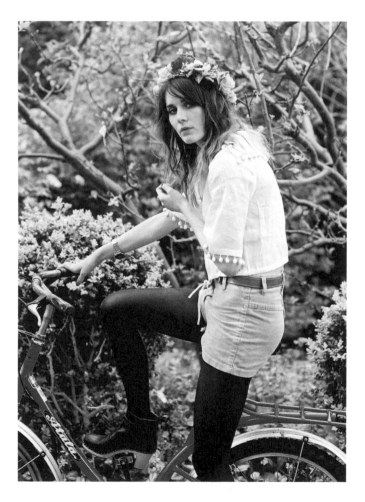

A former lawyer, Vanessa Jackman relocated from Sydney to London in mid-2007. Though she had never previously been interested in taking photographs, the new city opened up a world of inspiration to her and, picking up her husband's compact camera to document her new surroundings, Jackman began her enduring love affair with the shutter. Starting her blog in 2008 simply as a way of publishing these new images, Jackman rapidly earned a wide audience of readers who look to her for an effortless, classic take on style and beauty. Shooting both on the streets and at the world's most prestigious catwalk shows, Jackman's photographs, which are almost entirely of women, have found their way onto the pages of international fashion magazines and she has collaborated with a large number of high-profile websites and blogs. British, US and Australian *Vogue*, *Lucky* magazine, *W* magazine, *Harper's Bazaar* and both French and Russian *Glamour* have all included her imagery in editorials.

Below: Clémentine for *Grazia*
Opposite: Cara

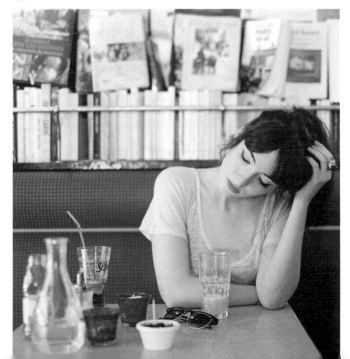

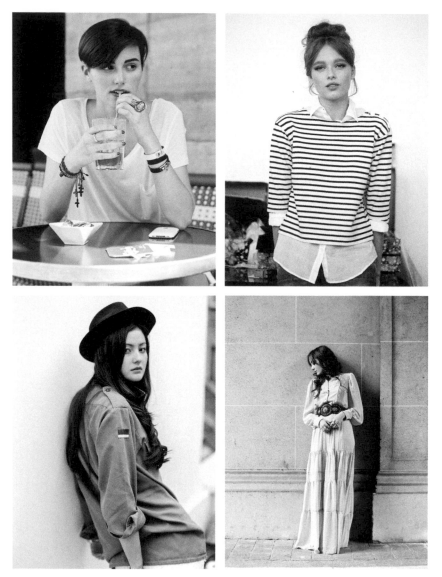

Top left: Anne-Catherine for *Grazia*, Paris
Top right: Beegee behind the scenes at MiH Jeans, S/S 2012
Bottom left: Peony
Bottom right: Louise for *Grazia*

Vanessa Jackman

'I started my blog as a way of keeping family and friends back home in Australia up to date with my photographic adventures. It has evolved into a portfolio featuring portraits, street style and travel images. I love to feature girls who inspire me with their style. For me, style is only partly about clothes. It encompasses so many things, like the way a person walks, smiles, laughs, wears their hair, how they accessorize, even small things like freckles or braces on their teeth. Those are the things that make a person unique and beautiful and are what I want to capture with my camera. I photograph what I love, what inspires me, and blog those images. I am not sure if that differentiates my blog from others - there are so many wonderful blogs out in the blogosphere - but mine is very "me", I guess, and hopefully that makes it unique.

I think blogging has opened many doors for people like me, who perhaps don't have a traditional background in fashion. Coming from a legal background, I didn't know anyone in the fashion industry before I started. The blog has given me wonderful opportunities that I doubt I would have had without it.'

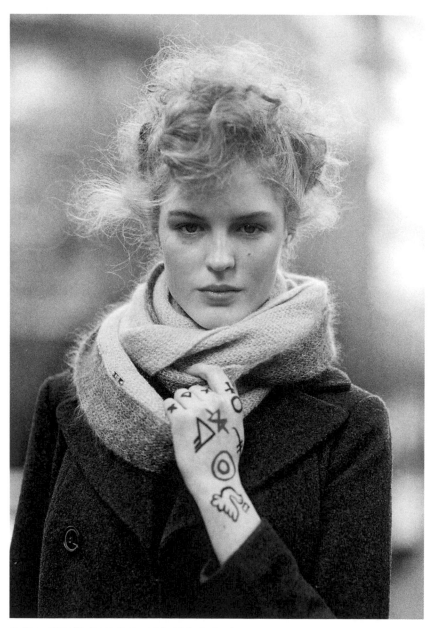

Bo Don, after Vivienne Westwood Red Label, London

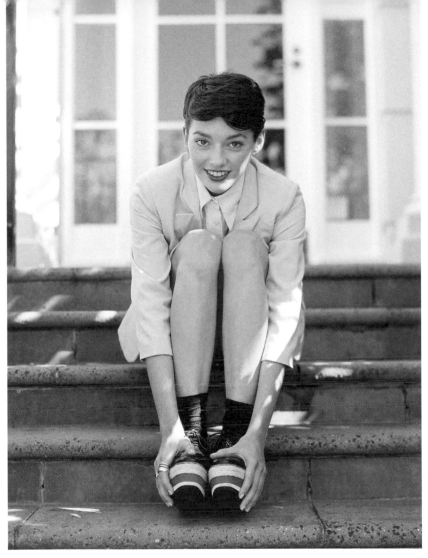

Renee Kitchen for *Grazia*

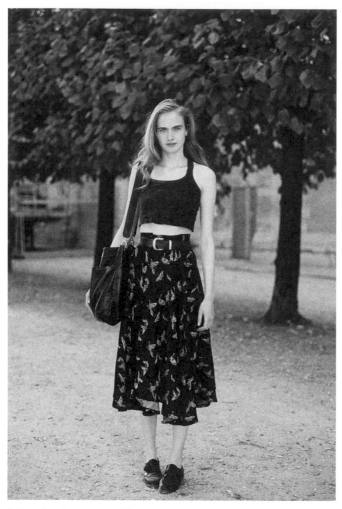

Butterflies for spring, after Léonard, Paris

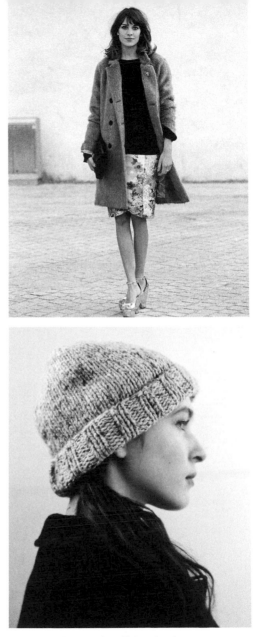

Top: Alexa Chung, after Erdem, London
Bottom: Backstage at Margaret Howell, London

Park & Cube

Shini Park

parkandcube.com

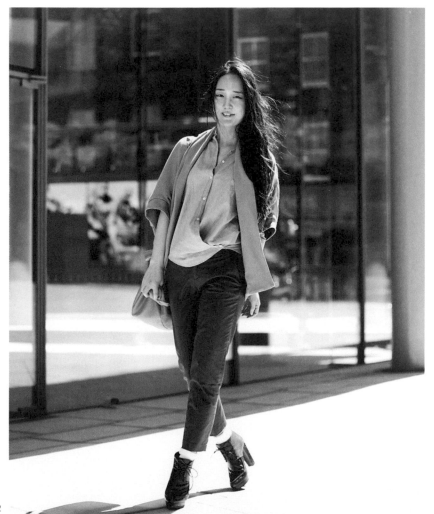

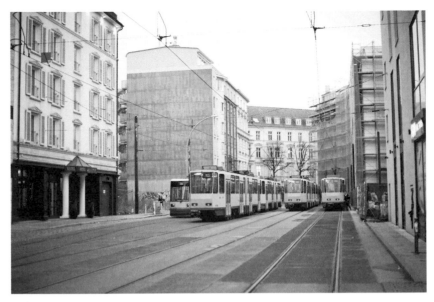

Berlin

Shini Park, a graphic design graduate from Central Saint Martins in London, set up Park & Cube in 2008 to provide an antidote to the more commercially minded, ratings-focused style blogs prevalent at the time. Park was all about the DIY, looking to give tips on designer alternatives alongside an insight into her own style. Picking up followers accordingly, Park & Cube's content has grown organically to become 'a lifestyle edit with lots of travel thrown in'. Touring regularly, mainly throughout Europe, the London-based Park provides a different take on fashion, looking more towards individual style or how to go about creating a unique look. A combination of high-street, vintage, DIY and choice finds holds her blog together, along with soft, beautifully washed-out images and idiosyncratic text. Now creative director at Editer.com and a contributor to *Vogue Brazil* and Glamour.com UK, Park has been deservedly recognized. The blog has led to collaborations with Guerlain, Patrizia Pepe and Pennyblack, and she is a brand ambassador for Guess.

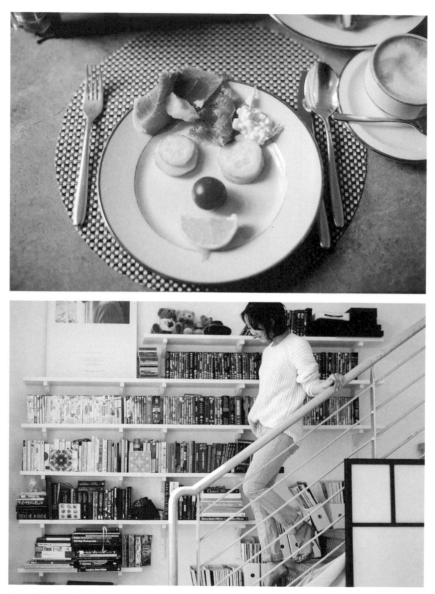

Top: Florence food

Shini Park

'My interest in blogging started to grow in the
few months after I discovered blogs with strong
identities. In time, I grew to dislike the idea
of giving a generic rating to supposedly "unique"
outfits, and the "buy buy buy" culture that was
increasingly popular on the new blogs. So I
decided, on a whim, to open my own space where
I could explore affordable fashion and DIY projects
and share style choices without feeling like
I'm in a popularity contest. The blog is a visual
diary reared mostly on my lifestyle and interests.
The posts might cover an unusual technique used
by a designer or a trend that could be replicable
with DIY.

I consider my blog to be a library of my personal
preferences; I try to make a point of only using
self-created content, mostly photography, to ensure
that readers won't see the same magazine clipping
they might have come across on another blog.

The biggest influence the blog has had on my work
is on my photography. There really is no better
lesson for an amateur photographer than to utilize
the camera every single day. It's also an outlet
to be creative at all times. I'm still a heavy
promoter of decency in dressing, and will always
strive to keep the content as unique as possible.'

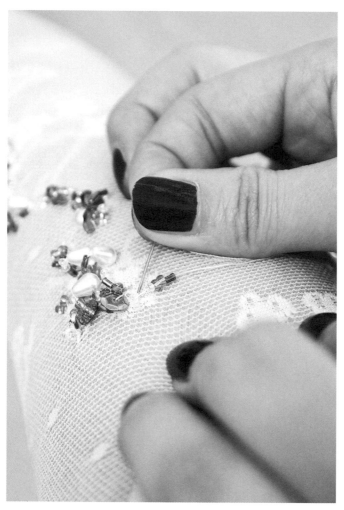

DIY beaded tights

DIY slashed jeans

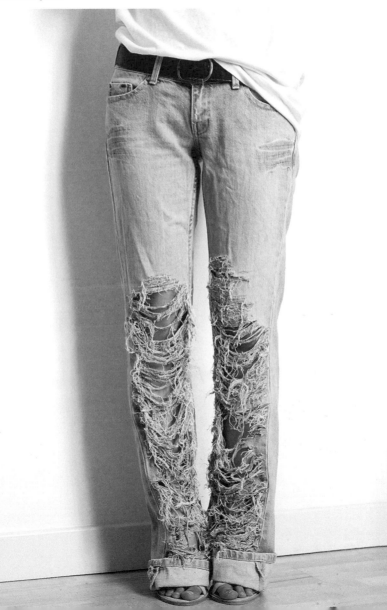

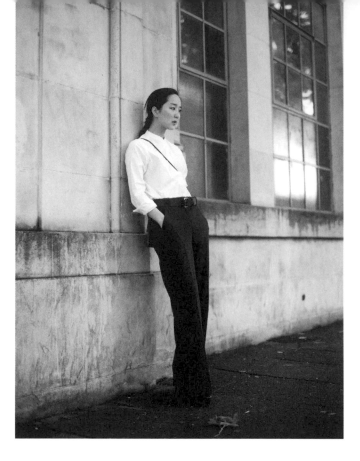

United Nude flagship store in Covent Garden, London

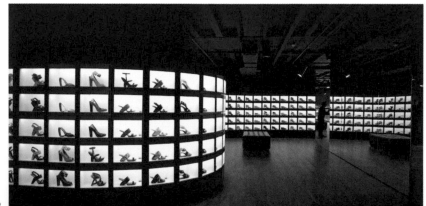

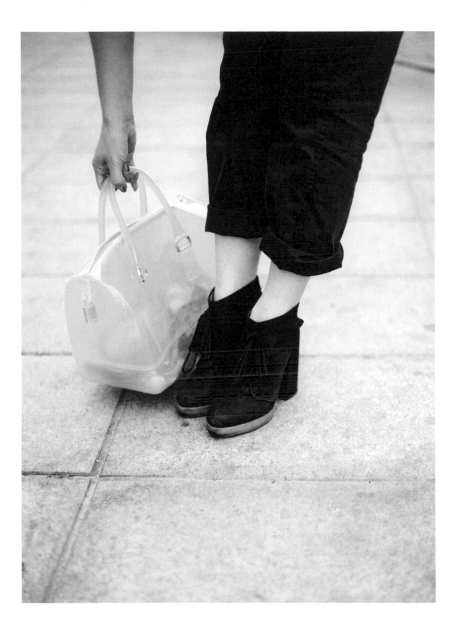

Buckets and Spades

Matthew Pike

buckets-and-spades.blogspot.co.uk

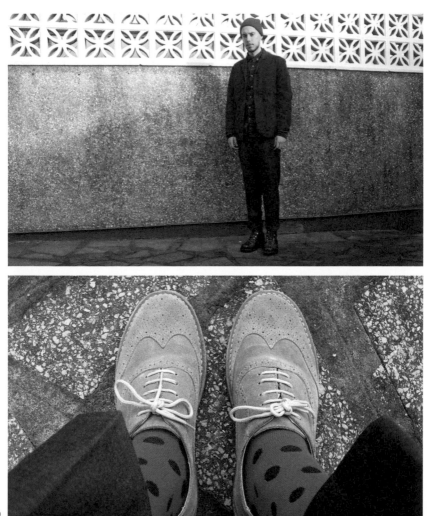

Blackpool-based blogger Matthew Pike takes a contemporary and relaxed attitude to menswear on Buckets and Spades, which he set up while studying fashion promotion at the University of Central Lancashire. After graduating in 2011 and now working in marketing and retail, Pike hunts for the detail in beautifully constructed clothes on his blog and is always interested in garments that have a handmade or British-made element. Describing his own style as a 'classic layered look', Buckets and Spades examines what he loves from the worlds of fashion, design, art and interiors. Alongside his personal posts, Pike provides a variety of imagery culled from different sources, highlighting his interests in graphics, colour, signage and details.

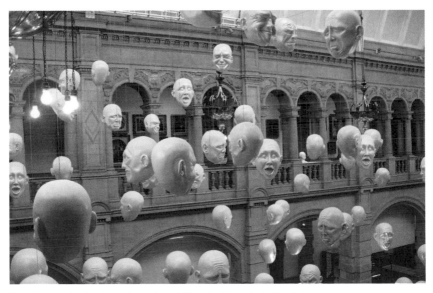

Floating heads dangling from the ceiling in the main hall of the Kelvingrove Museum, Glasgow, installation by Sophy Cave

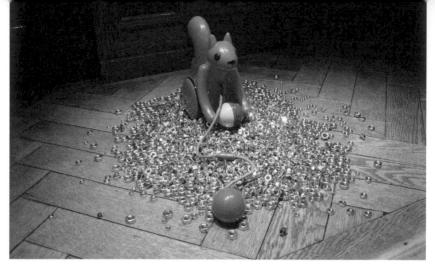

Display in Paul Smith's window on Floral St, London

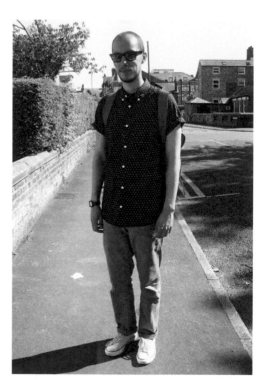

Matthew Pike

'I feature a lot of designers and brands that
use colour, creative set design, typography
and graphics. I feature stuff I really love
or it might just be a certain colour combination
that someone used on packaging or an old sign.
It's these design decisions that really interest
me, why they chose to go with a certain colour, cut
and fabric. I also like to feature local artists
and community causes. I read a lot of blogs from
around the UK and their writers are always visiting
new galleries, museums, restaurants, shops and
areas that I would not otherwise know about.
This really inspires what I do and a lot of the
time I will make a note of these places and try
to visit them.

I'm very inspired by old America – the working
class, youth cultures, music and art movements
– but on the flip side I'm really interested in
technology advancements, architecture, homeware
and interiors. I would say my aesthetic is modern,
but heavily influenced by the past.

Blogging means that everybody can have a voice
now. It has made sharing as easy as it's ever been;
independent brands and small designers get great
exposure from it.'

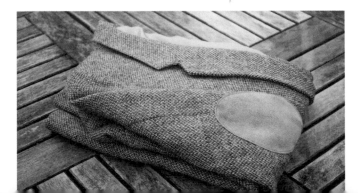

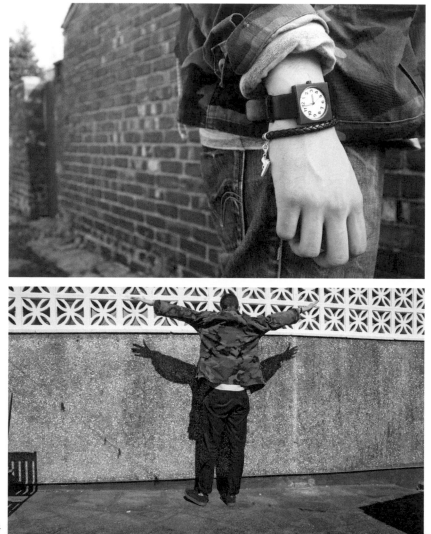

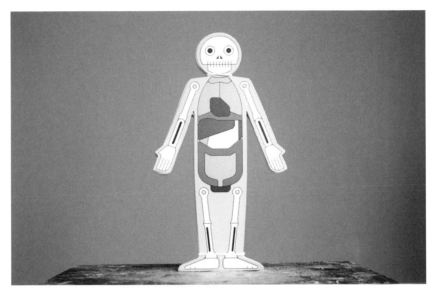

Muji human body puzzle

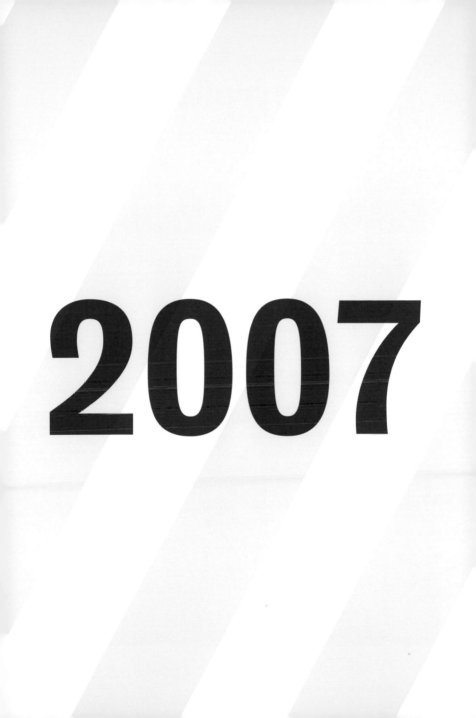

2007

Disneyrollergirl

Navaz Batliwalla

disneyrollergirl.net

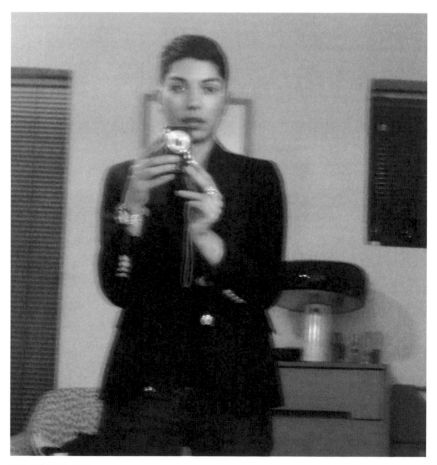

Navaz Batliwalla

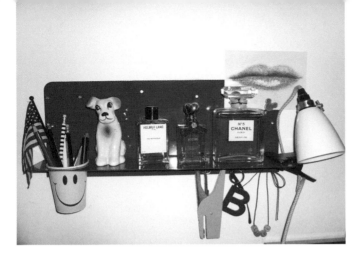

Initially starting her blog to be free of commercial publishing's restraints, London-based industry insider Navaz Batliwalla began Disneyrollergirl anonymously in 2007. While working as the fashion director of *CosmoGirl!* and as a freelance writer for Handbag.com, Batliwalla felt that some of her personal opinions were restricted and sought a new channel of communication. Rapidly garnering a huge following of both interested members of the public and high-profile fans, after four years, in 2011, she came out of hiding, announcing her identity publicly through the site. Now in the public eye, Batliwalla uses Disneyrollergirl to comment on the fast-paced industry and the changes happening across the landscape because of the advent of digital publishing. 'I can be a writer, a stylist, a buyer and a publisher and still remain completely independent', she asserts. The blog combines conversations with those working behind the scenes with descriptions of Batliwalla's personal style choices and the events she attends. Now lecturing and working creatively with a number of brands, including Ralph Lauren, H&M, Harvey Nichols and Browns, Batliwalla uses all her skills on the blog to create an all-encompassing outlet for her work and ideas.

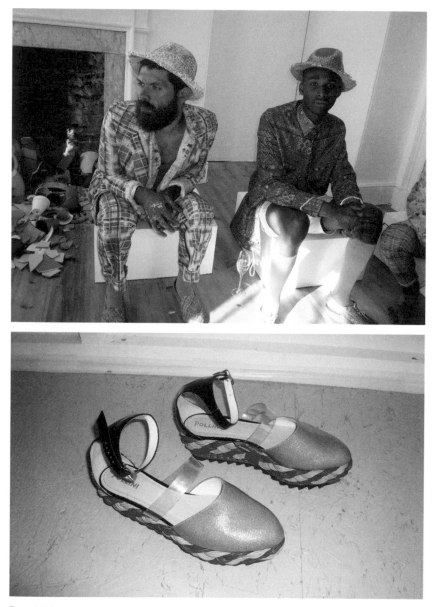

Top: Agi & Sam, A/W 11 collection
Bottom: Louise Gray shoes, S/S 12

Navaz Batliwalla

'One of the biggest highlights has been
developing an interest in and understanding
of the online fashion world. I have met some
pioneering and fascinating digital innovators
and really enjoy talking to them about the future
of fashion, design and digital media. I have
always kept scrapbooks and diaries so I liked
the idea of blogging being a bit rough and ready,
like a fanzine. I don't really have an agenda:
Disneyrollergirl is completely self-indulgent.
I always say it's a place to empty my brain. My
personal aesthetic is mostly unisex, comfortable,
utilitarian and classic. I'm a people-watcher
so I like to notice elements of a person's style
and sometimes I'll appropriate it for myself.
I'm always looking at artists from the 1960s –
I like the crumpled, casual look of Hockney,
Rauschenberg and Warhol but with finesse. Also
The Clash and the Buffalo kids from the 1980s
and all the androgynous i-D girls from that time.
But I love quality and luxury too so I think it's
a mixture.

I try not to put pictures of myself on the blog;
coming from a magazine background, I know all
about giving the reader more value. I like
there to be a surprise, so I really work hard
to vary the posts, put something funny or silly
next to something serious, mention an obscure
photographer or make unexpected connections
between seemingly random ideas.

The industry is changing. Bloggers have helped
open up access to designers and to fashion and
the consequence is that people want to dress
up, experiment, be part of it.'

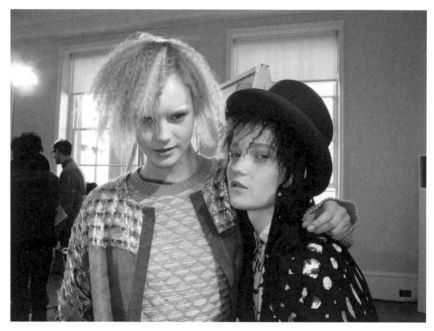

At Louise Gray catwalk show, A/W 10

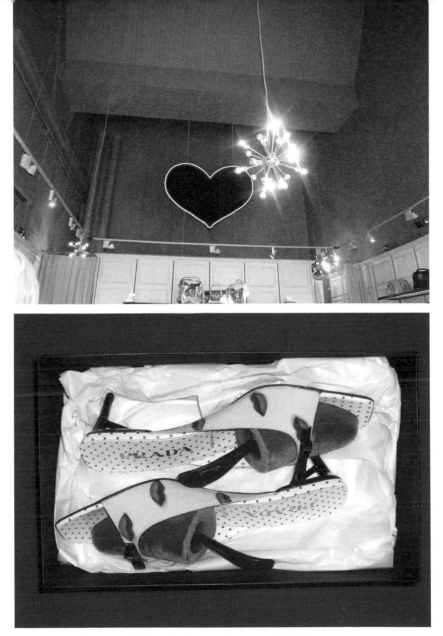

Top: Luella at Bicester Village for British Designers Collective
boutique, Oxfordshire

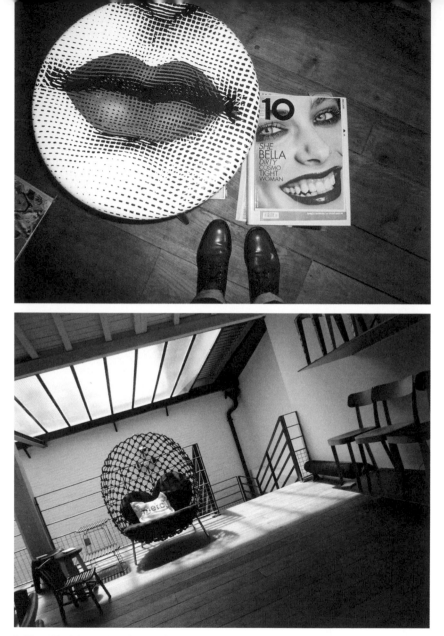

Bottom: Inside charity-focused luxury concept boutique Merci, Paris

Quentin Jones's installation at Darkroom, London

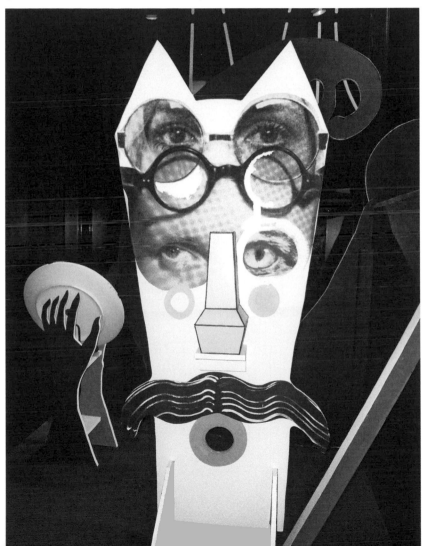

Kate Loves Me

Pelayo Diaz

katelovesme.net

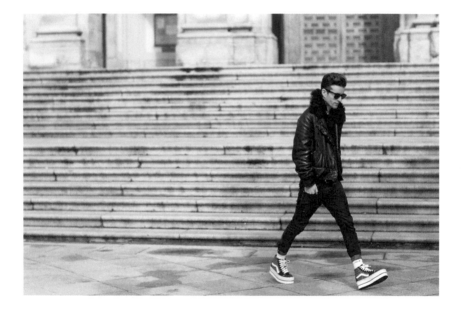

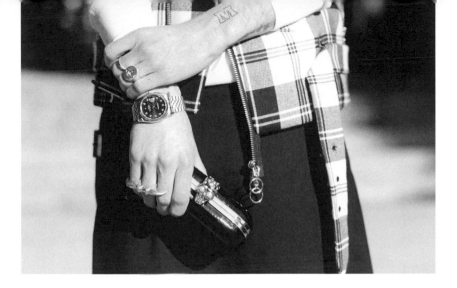

After moving from Madrid to London to study fashion at Central St Martins, and while interning at Giles Deacon and McQ, Pelayo Diaz, better known as Prince Pelayo, decided to start blogging about the exciting life he was leading. Covering backstage at fashion shows, parties, people and his own style, he started Kate Loves Me in 2007, initially as a way of showing his friends and family at home what he was getting up to. The blog rapidly earned itself a following of readers yearning to get a glimpse of the prince's glamorous existence. Since being featured in magazines and on websites and blogs worldwide, including *Vogue Korea*, *L'Officiel Hommes China*, *GQ*, *WAD* magazine, Bryanboy and The Sartorialist, Diaz has garnered himself a place in the blogging inner circle. His individual look is very much London-inspired, with a rock sensibility teamed with high-end design. Givenchy, Prada, leather biker jackets and a 1950s quiff are all elements of his signature style. Diaz has also modelled for a number of designers, produces his own capsule line and has collaborated with Spanish designer Davidelfin on accessories.

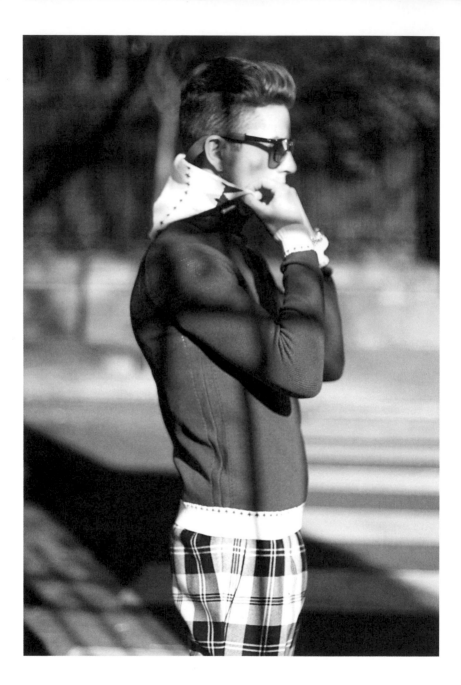

Pelayo Diaz

'I wanted to share my first impressions of life
in London with people back in Spain, as they were
always curious about what I was doing. I needed
a platform where I could upload pictures and write
longer texts, so I started blogging. I've always
loved writing, I have kept journals daily since
I was 13, so I guess the blog was just a more fun,
2.0 version of them. At the beginning it was more
about my feelings and my day-to-day life, but
as you gain followers there are things you don't
feel like sharing anymore. I guess now it's more
editorial, more visually elaborate. What I cover
now is a small part of my life, but I love fashion
so that has to show somehow – hence the many
self-portraits of me wearing my favourite pieces
every season.

I have to connect with the designer or the trend
– I have to see some part of me in them, whether
real or not. I think my job is not just about the
clothes, but also about the journey to find them.

London has made a huge scar on my style, in
a good way of course. I never look too serious;
there is a young-boy factor that I try never
to lose. If you look around at the people that
make up the fashion industry, the majority look
as though they are not enjoying it. Bloggers are
there because they want to be: because they
enjoy every second, every glance.'

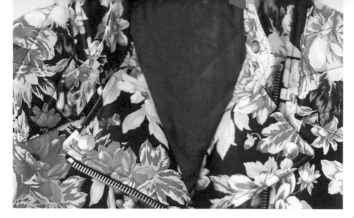

Above: Céline floral biker jacket, S/S 12

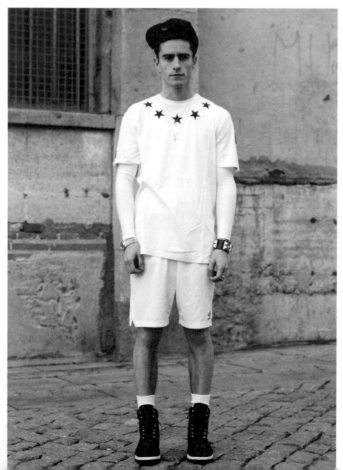

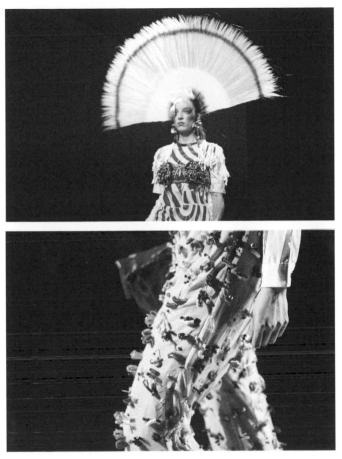

Top & bottom: Louise Gray, A/W 12, London Fashion Week

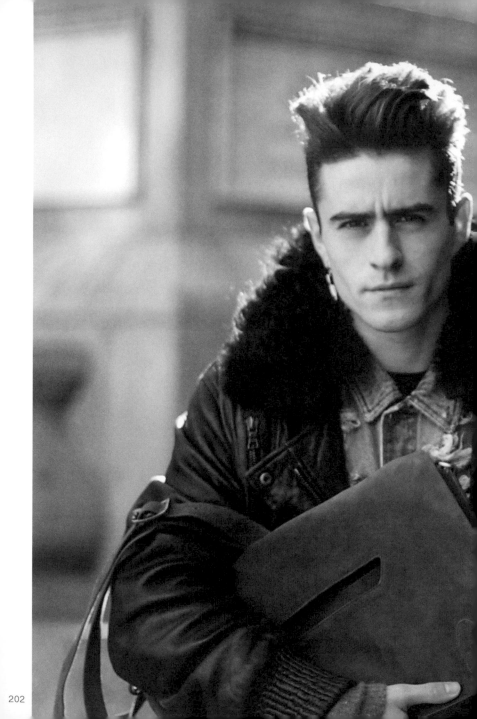

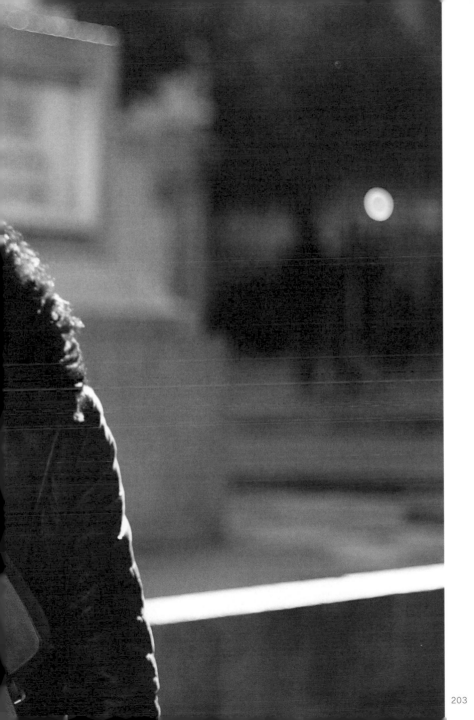

The Business of Fashion

Imran Amed

businessoffashion.com

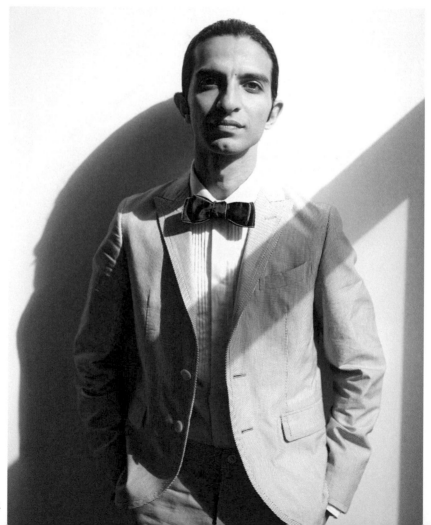

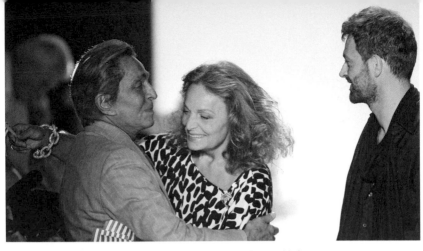

Above: Valentino with Diane Von Furstenberg at her Spring 2012
fashion show during Mercedes-Benz Fashion Week in New York City
Opposite: Imran Amed

Previously working as a management consultant at global firm
McKinsey & Co., Canadian-born Imran Amed set up The Business
of Fashion in 2007 from the comfort of his London home. Described
as a 'daily destination for fashion's most influential power
players' by AnOther Magazine and 'indispensable for the
multi-billion dollar industry' by lifestyle website Nowness,
BoF is considered a leading platform for news and insight into
the luxury and fashion markets. Steering clear of style
inspiration or recommendations, Amed's focus is on the world
behind the products and the ever-changing roles of those
working in the industry. Read by creatives, executives, students
and entrepreneurs in over 200 countries and territories around
the world, the author's expertise is regularly called upon
by the international fashion and business media, including CNN,
the BBC, the New York Times, the Wall Street Journal and Women's
Wear Daily. He is an expert advisor to board-level executives
at leading luxury and fashion brands, judges prestigious
design competitions internationally, is an associate lecturer
at Central St Martins College of Art & Design and sits on
the board of the British Fashion Council Digital and Menswear
2012 committees.

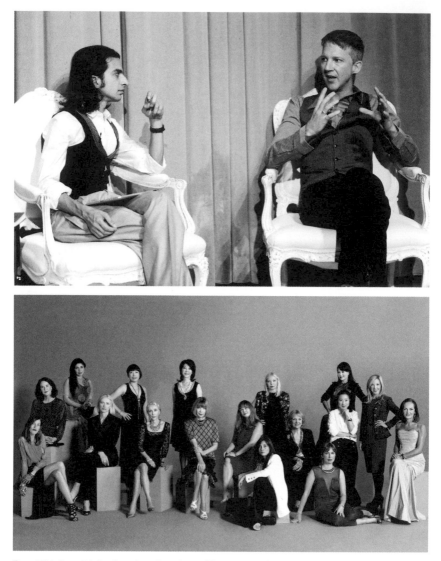

Top: With *Dazed & Confused* co-founder Jefferson Hack for BoF Fashion Pioneers
Bottom: *Vogue* editors from around the world

Imran Amed

'I was looking for a creative outlet to explore
my budding interest in the fashion industry
and I noticed that nobody was writing about
the business of fashion itself. Many business
publications focused on fashion are not all that
worried about aesthetics. I learned early on
that in our industry, aesthetics count for a lot.
In fact, if things aren't designed and presented
well, people won't pay attention to the words and
content, no matter how intelligent, interesting
or exciting they may be.

We love to tell good stories of personal and
professional triumphs and successes but also
of the errors and misjudgements along the
way. We cover the inner workings of the fashion
industry at the intersection of creativity,
business and digital platforms. We have a global
outlook and point of view, and we engage our
audience in discussion. We show the industry
in a different light from the mainstream focus
on glamour and the glossy surface of fashion.

BoF has opened a world of new opportunities
for me and our team of editors and contributors
all around the globe. It helps to bring us in
touch with the people who are shaping the fashion
industry today. Fashion blogging has added
a new set of individual voices to fashion, voices
that were not previously heard. It has helped
to demystify an industry that was initially very
closed off.'

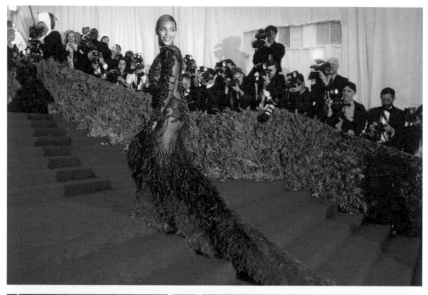

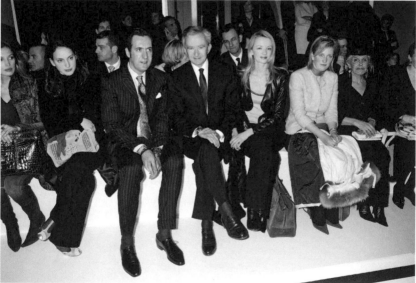

Top: Beyoncé attends the Costume Institute Gala Benefit at The Metropolitan Museum of Art in New York City
Bottom: Princess Olga Isabelle, Jaime de Marichalar, Bernard Arnault, Delphine Arnault and Princess Astrid of Belgium at Paris Fashion Week

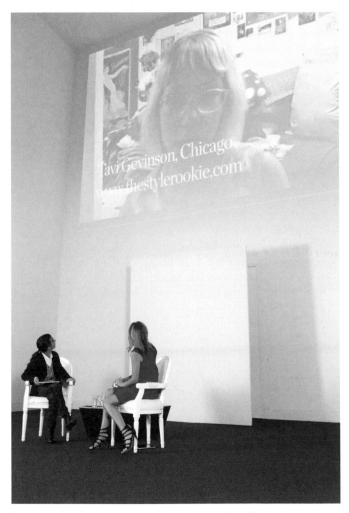

BoF meets Net-A-Porter and Mr Porter founder Natalie Massenet
and Tavi Gevinson, on screen

Fashionista

Leah Chernikoff - executive editor
Cheryl Wischhover - features and beauty editor
Hayley Phelan - news editor
Dhani Mau - associate editor

fashionista.com

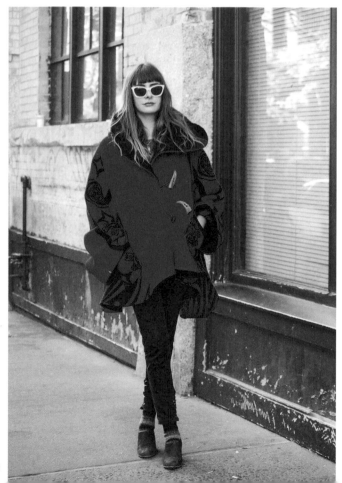

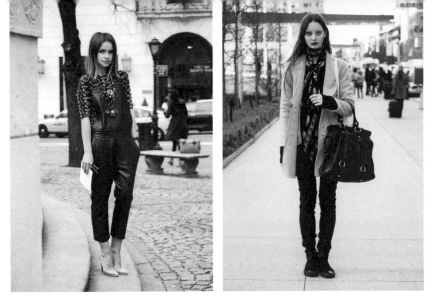

Left: Miroslava
Right: Codie
Opposite: Lindsey

Fashionista is one of the few independent websites that
have the accessible approach of blogging, the freedom to be
opinionated and the speed to be able to comment on industry
news immediately. Based in New York, it has four full-time
editors who work alongside an army of contacts and contributors
to provide up-to-the-minute information. By retaining its
commercial independence, the site has been able to grow and
evolve organically, sharing commentary that is not guided
by an affiliation with a particular brand or company. The ways
in which people access fashion design and creative content
are no longer restricted to the pages of magazines or gallery
walls, and foresighted blogs that grow in the way Fashionista
has provide an important model for the future of publishing.

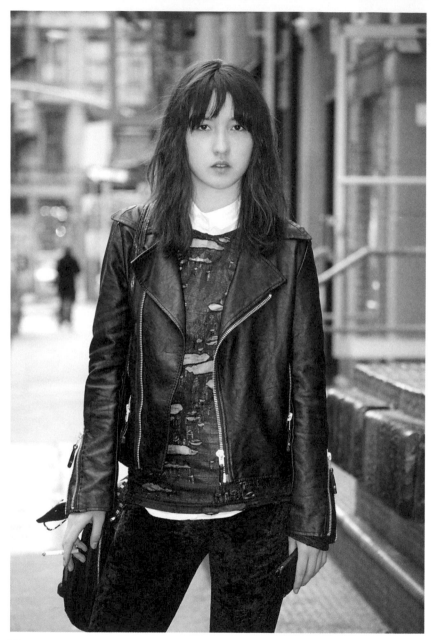

Nina

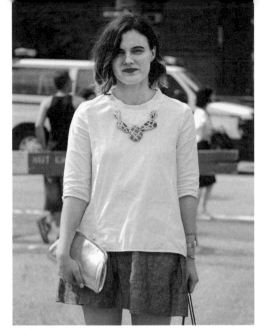

Julia

Leah Chernikoff

'I came to Fashionista from the New York *Daily News* because I wanted to gain experience in the digital realm and continue to report on fashion. It was easy to see that the media were moving online and I wanted to figure out how it all worked! We're news-driven: whenever a designer or brand makes news, anyway! That could mean anything from a gimmicky runway show, like sending out a custom-made train on the runway *à la* Louis Vuitton, to a celebrity designing a collection, see Kanye West, or simply a designer presenting a fantastic forward-thinking collection, like Raf Simons for Jil Sander. We're one of a handful of independent fashion news sites; this gives us the freedom to report on almost whatever we want and be silly whenever we want. A sense of humour is key!'

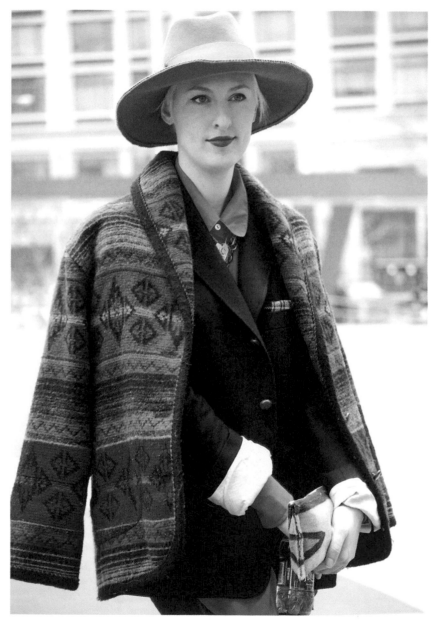

Lisa

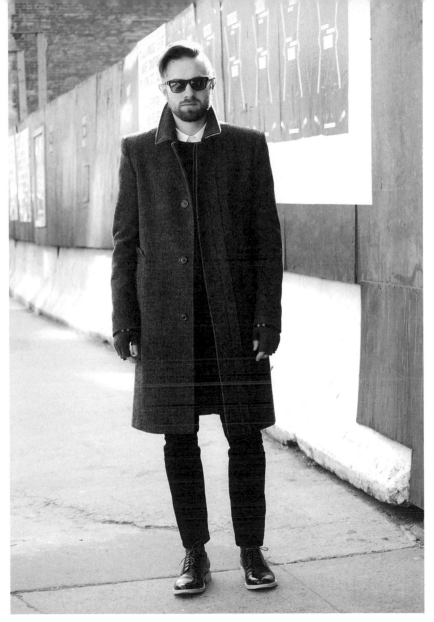

Nicholas

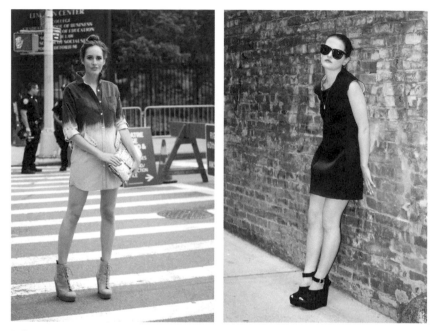

Left: Louise
Right: Lizzy

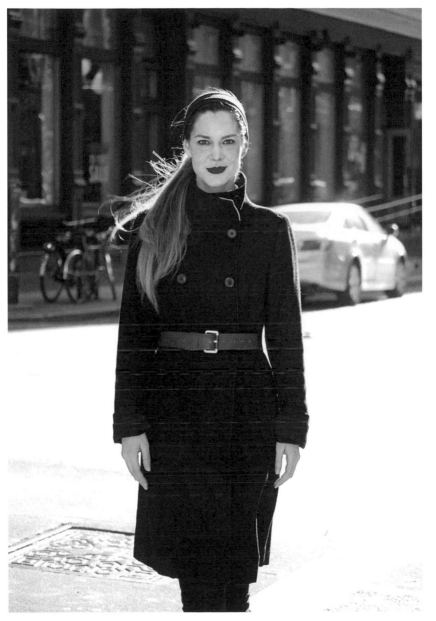

Gayle

Amlul

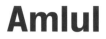

Gala Gonzalez

amlul.com

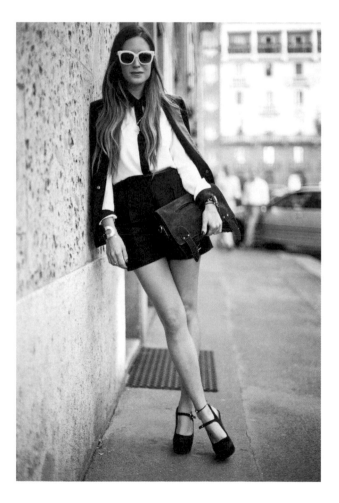

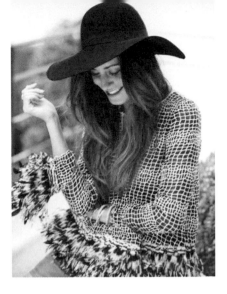

After graduating from the London College of Fashion and Central St Martins with a focus on fashion design and promotion, Gala Gonzalez set up Amlul in 2007. Seriously web-savvy, Gonzalez has used the portal to share her voice, reaching an international network of readers and successfully launching a career as an 'It Girl'. Her blog centres on self-styled portrait posts, photos from parties and events that she has attended, brand campaigns and editorials she has modelled for and behind-the-scenes reportage. Amlul has been featured in over 100 publications around the globe, including *Vogue*, *Elle*, *Marie Claire* and *Teen Vogue*, and Gonzalez makes regular appearances on the pages of society and style magazines worldwide. Hers is very much an 'ego-blog', as she herself says, but one in which the reader is invited to join in her excitement. Hers is a strong example of the career that a blogger can build, as Gonzalez has subsequently worked with Louis Vuitton, Zara and Elie Saab, modelled in campaigns for Loewe, Diesel, Mango, Corello and H&M, and become a contributor to *Vogue Spain*.

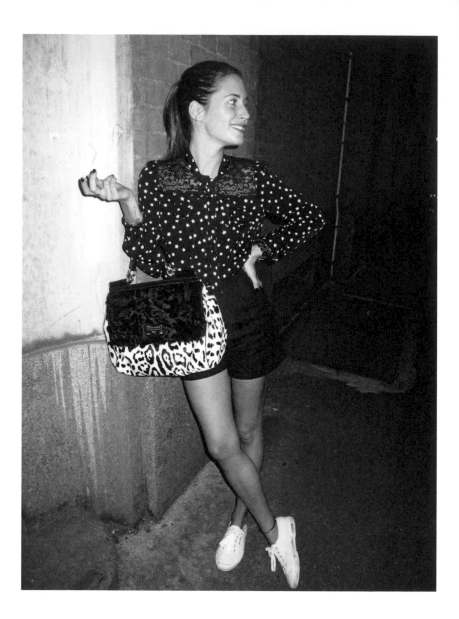

Gala Gonzalez

'The newspaper *El País* published my original Fotolog visual diary as one of the influential sites coming from Spain and from there I decided to focus purely on fashion, as I was just starting to study it. My posts always somehow have to reflect my style and mood. I don't talk about things or trends just for the sake of it; they have to be relevant to my readers. I'm very eclectic and very bohemian, I would have loved to attend Woodstock and to have met Jim Morrison. I don't believe much in the now, but I don't want to live in the past.

I believe in the modern woman, so for me it is important that women feel confident without the need to show their cleavage. Dressing is our initial business card: others are going to perceive what we want to communicate. Amlul has become like some sort of public display window through which people can see what I am doing, behind the camera. For most of my readers that don't live in big cities, Amlul allows them to follow the fashion adventure through my eyes.'

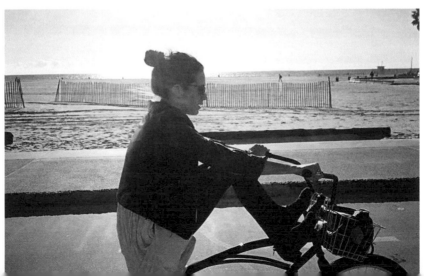

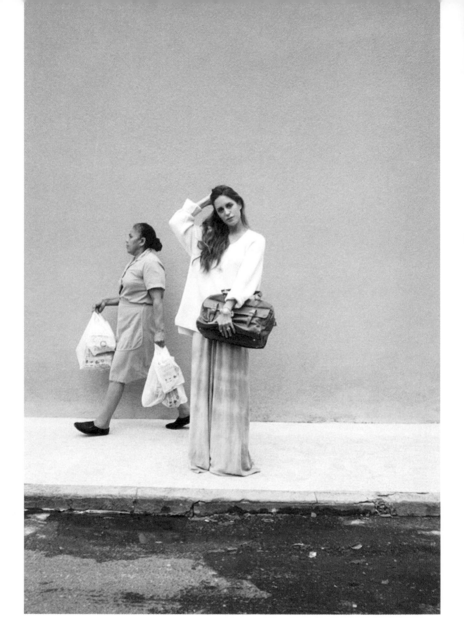

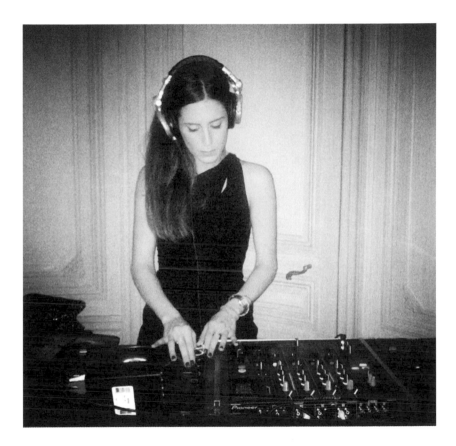

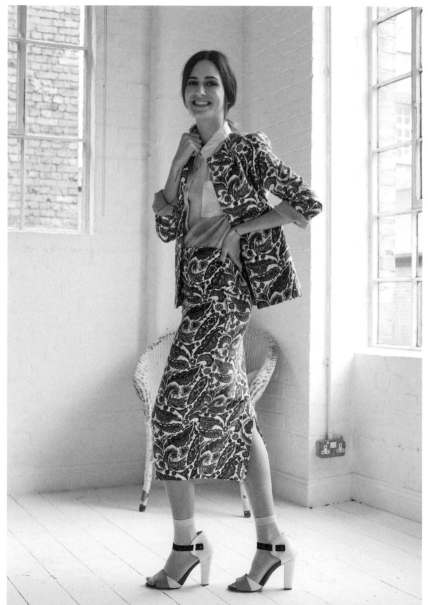

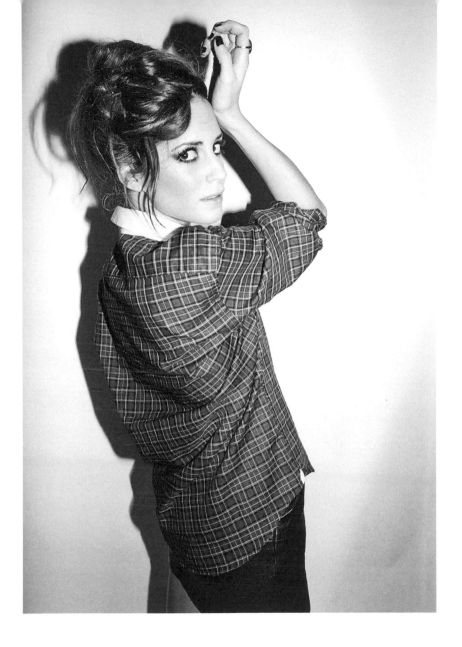

Style Salvage

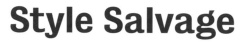

Steve Salter and EJ
stylesalvage.blogspot.co.uk

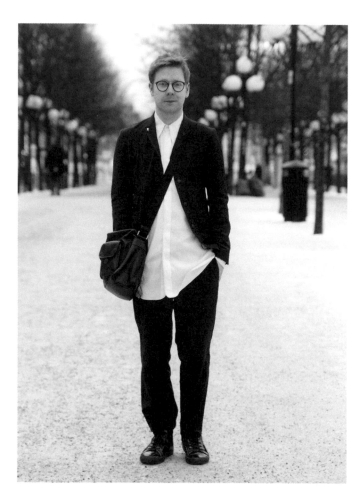

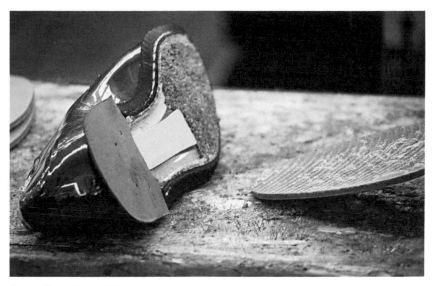

Above: The making of Cheaney brogues
Opposite: Steve Salter

Devised as an open discussion between friends Steve Salter
and EJ, based in London and Manchester respectively, Style
Salvage is a menswear blog with a sharp focus on 'how
men could and do dress'. Set up in 2007, it has developed from
a very personal hobby into a platform that has brought the
duo into contact with the designers and industry insiders
about whom they write. The blog's aesthetic centres on
tailoring, classic shapes and technical construction across
emerging and established designers and heritage brands. The
Style Salvage team has developed a voice that is knowledgeable
but does not isolate its readership. It is not a blog that looks
to present an unattainable or idealistic code of dressing,
but one that democratizes style. The site's posts are split
into style commentary, seven-day style diaries and interviews
with designers, journalists and shop-owners, mixed in with the
occasional easy DIY project and personal style shot. It allows
its readers into the world of two people obsessed by clothes
that are equally creative and wearable.

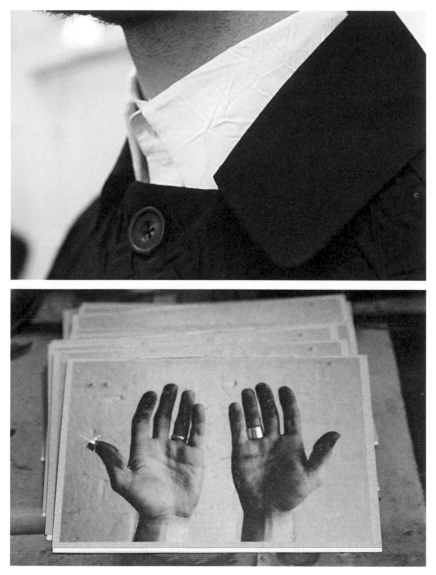

Top: Christopher O'Brien, A/W 12
Bottom: Sebastian Tarek studio visit

Steve Salter

'We spent a great deal of time with each other at university. Whenever the student loan came in, we always made a dash to the shops. While I was working in London and she in Manchester, we spent far too much of our time sending each other procrastinating emails containing everything from bargain finds to high-street releases, Fred Astaire's style tips and Stockholm street style snaps. We have always discussed men's style, and one day we just thought: why not start a blog together? The blog aims to showcase emerging and established design talent whilst exuding a penchant for quality, tailoring and a general openness to self-expression. Over the last few years we have built up strong links with the designers we love and we try and feature them in a new way each season. We like nothing more than hearing about a designer's inspiration and following their creative processes right through to the finished pieces.

The growing influence of blogging and the seemingly relentless pace of the Internet has changed how we consume more traditional forms of fashion media. I think we will see magazines continue to evolve from the throwaway monthly model to much more limited and special releases, issues that we will cherish for years as opposed to minutes!'

Mr Hare in Mr Hare Hannibal XI blacks and Levi's

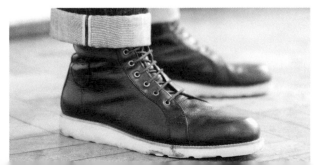

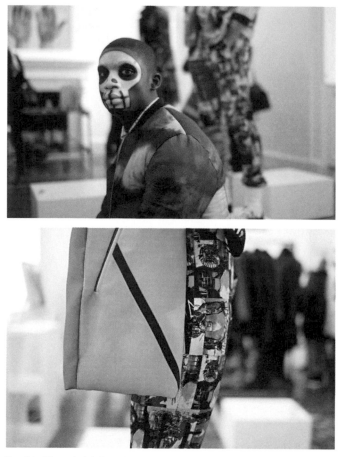

Top & bottom: Agi & Sam, A/W 12

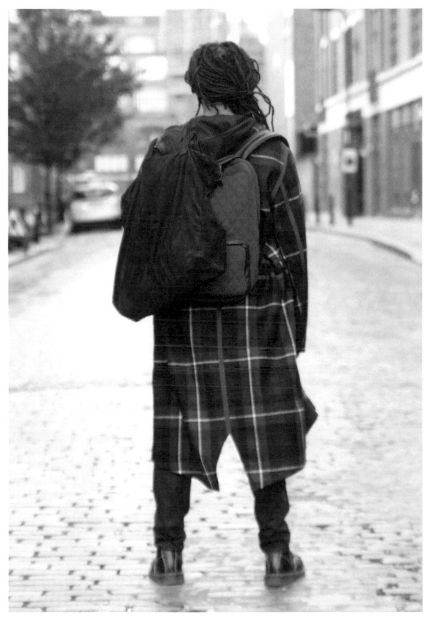

Style stalking … Harris Elliott

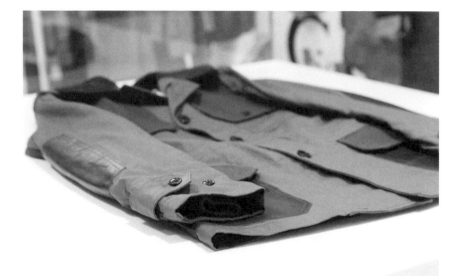

A visit to Goodhood: Junya Watanabe man parka

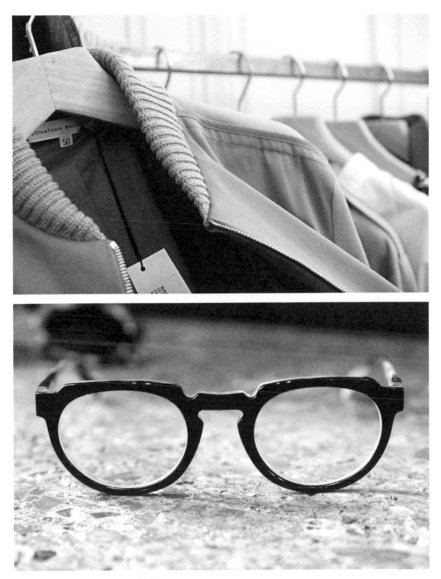

Top: Jonathan Saunders, S/S 12
Bottom: The showroom next door, A/W 12 ... Bruno Chaussignand

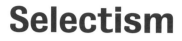

Selectism

Jeff Carvalho

selectism.com

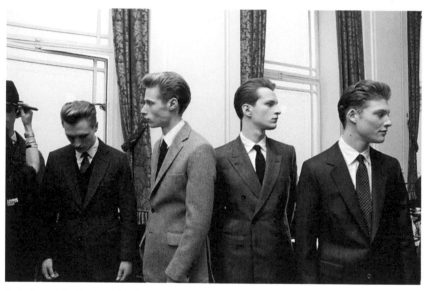

Backstage | E. Tautz, A/W 12

The former host of WeeklyDrop, a podcast dedicated to footwear and lifestyle, Jeff Carvalho set up Selectism in 2007 after a conversation with David Fischer, founder of HighSnobiety. With similar views on menswear, streetwear, design and art, and thoughts on how the HighSnobiety model could be taken in new directions, the pair decided that Carvalho should spearhead a new brand as part of the family. Now one of the most read sites on these subjects, Selectism provides a destination for men looking to 'explore and discover' the worlds of fashion, accessories, art, design, cars and travel, as Carvalho puts it. The point of reference for Selectism is always a certain feeling of luxury and obsession; desirable pieces to yearn after. Fashion is very much the differentiation between Selectism and the rest of the HighSnobiety group. It is a place for the discerning man who is just as excited by process and heritage as he is by the latest high-end designer. Initially focusing on clothing and footwear, the site has evolved in keeping with the tastes of its readership. 'We now offer much wider coverage, as our audience has asked for it and we plan to give it to them', says Carvalho. Selectism provides fashion and culturally relevant lifestyle information in a simple, clean form that allows the excitement of its contributors to shine through.

Store Visit | LN-CC

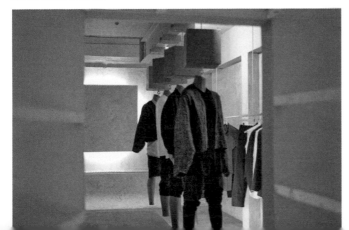

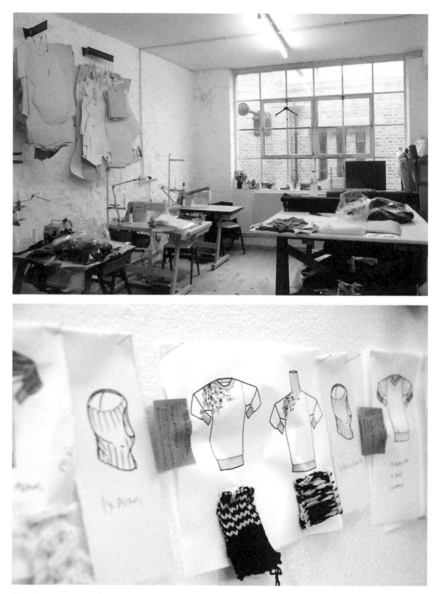

Top: Studio Visit | Lou Dalton
Bottom: Lou Dalton A/W 12 jumper design prototypes

Jeff Carvalho

'Our focus is primarily on providing readers
with information on what's new on the market.
This is what we do best. Risk and relevance are
the two things we look for in a designer. We read
and refer to a wide variety of sites, both within
fashion and outside it, and we are definitely
inspired by what others are discovering, making
note of it when it fits. Blogging has brought a huge
headache to some and a clear way to communicate
to a receptive audience to others. Fashion houses
are embracing the reach and influence that many
bloggers have, but this is not a one-size-fits-all
solution. On HighSnobiety, the content that we
cover has changed as our audience has grown.
The same is true of Selectism.'

Lou Dalton A/W 12 collection

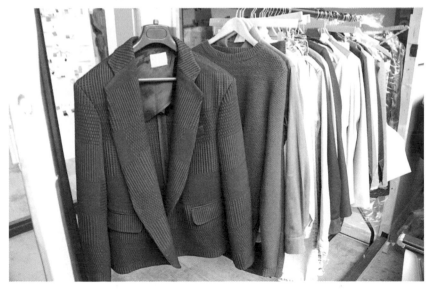

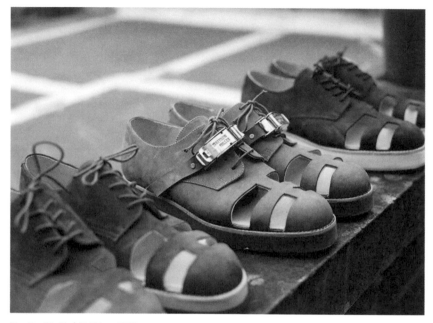

Studio Visit | Matthew Miller

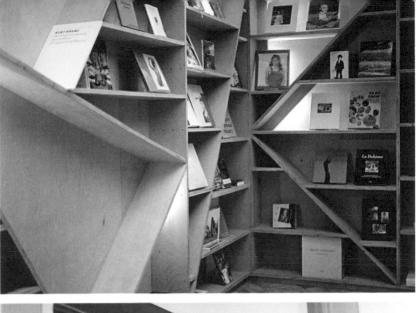

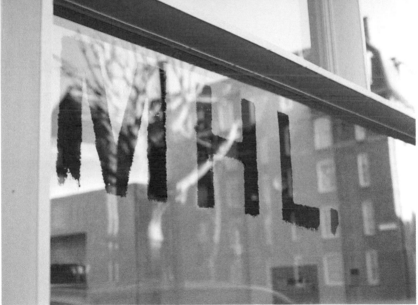

Top: Store Visit | LN-CC
Bottom: Store Visit | MHL, Margaret Howell, London

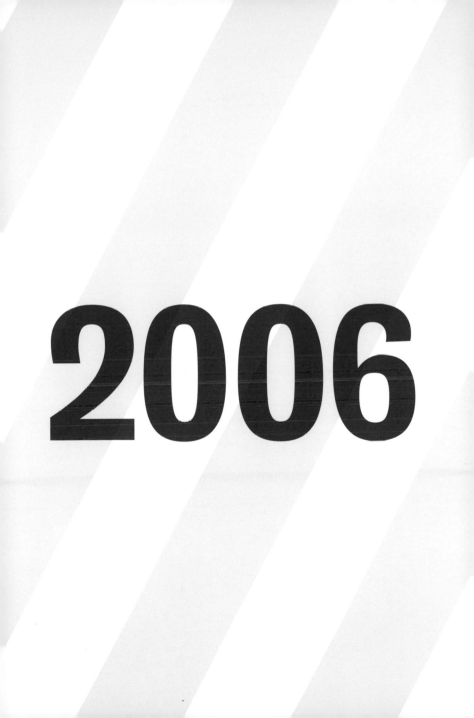

2006

Un Nouveau Ideal

Filep Motwary

unnouveauideal.typepad.com

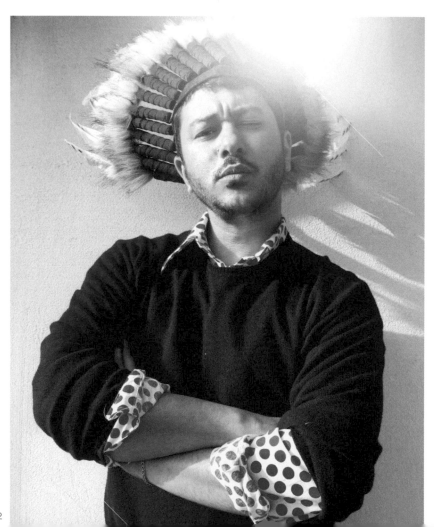

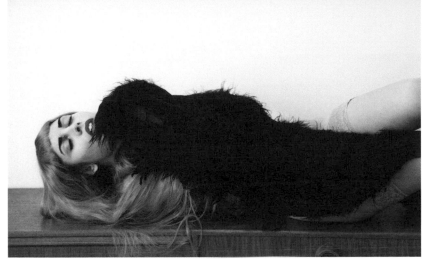

Above: C.T. (model) for Joanna Louca Woven Accessories, A/W 12/13
Opposite: Filep Motwary

Truly inspired by fashion design and based in both Nicosia, Cyprus, and Paris, Filep Motwary, photographer, editor and designer, is well-versed in all facets of the industry. He has a background that includes internships at John Galliano, Dior Couture and Chloé and a role as assistant stylist for *L'Officiel* in Greece, followed by four years as first assistant designer at Loukia Couture, Athens. After contributing regularly to Diane Pernet's blog A Shaded View on Fashion, in 2006 the Cypriot-Syrian Motwary, who studied fashion in both Milan and Athens, decided to start his own site, Un Nouveau Ideal. The effortlessly chic blog examines all the areas of culture that interest the author, communicating his personal aesthetic and inspirations through interviews with and features on a host of leading and emerging designers and artists. Using his industry connections, Motwary has posted conversations with iconic figures including Dries Van Noten, Helmut Lang, Yohji Yamamoto, Juergen Teller, Hans Feurer, Rick Owens and Christian Lacroix. He also works as the fashion features editor of *Dapper Dan* magazine, co-edited by Nicholas Georgiou and Vassilis Karidis. Un Nouveau Ideal is an invaluable resource focused on the fashion world and its various incarnations.

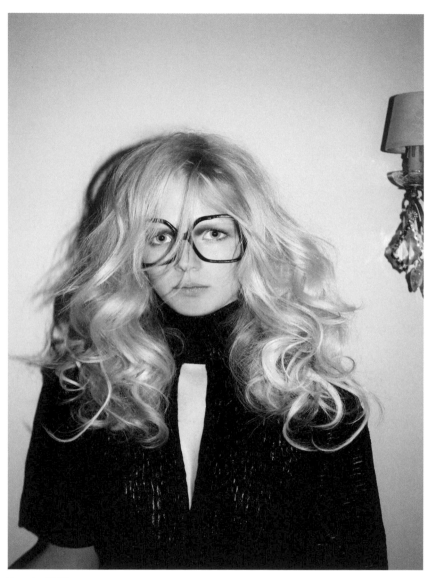

Hannah, 2008

Filep Motwary

'I was a contributor for Diane Pernet and things
reached a point where I felt I had to move in my
own direction. In the beginning I couldn't really
decide in which direction Un Nouveau Ideal would
go. Time gave me good experience and through it
I discovered many other possibilities apart from
fashion design. As a child, I was always asking
so many questions that people around me would get
irritated. As an adult, I interview the people that
really interest me; I like talking but despise
conversation for the sake of conversation. So far
I have spoken to many legends, but there are still
people I want to interview, like Cathy Horyn or
Serge Lutens. I regret not interviewing Alexander
McQueen and Isabella Blow.

It is the detail and the vision that inspires
me to feature people on Un Nouveau Ideal. I truly
understand fashion, the craft, the struggle
a designer and the team goes through when creating,
because I have been there and still am. When I see
a collection, it becomes obvious whether there
is a concept or not, whether the collection will
sell or not and to whom. If it's a young designer,
the rules are still the same. Why should one
person's work be more important than another's?
Although there are no rules on what Un Nouveau
Ideal is really about, somehow its profile and aim
are pretty clear.'

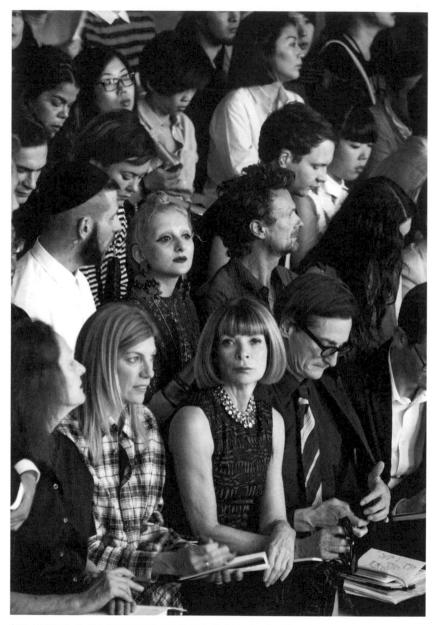

Anna Wintour, Grace Coddington and Hamish Bowles at a fashion show

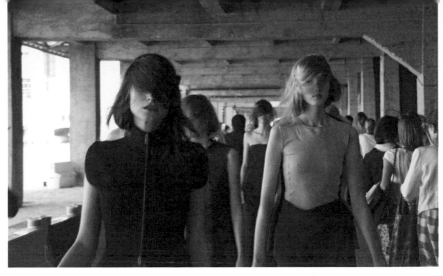

Top: Models at the Maison Martin Margiela show, S/S 12
Bottom: Yohji Yamamoto

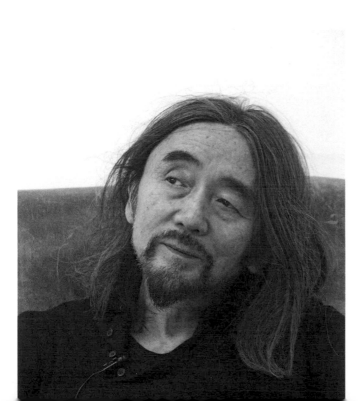

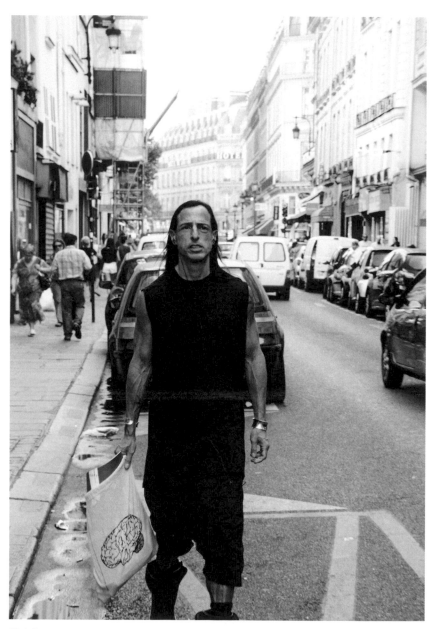

Rick Owens

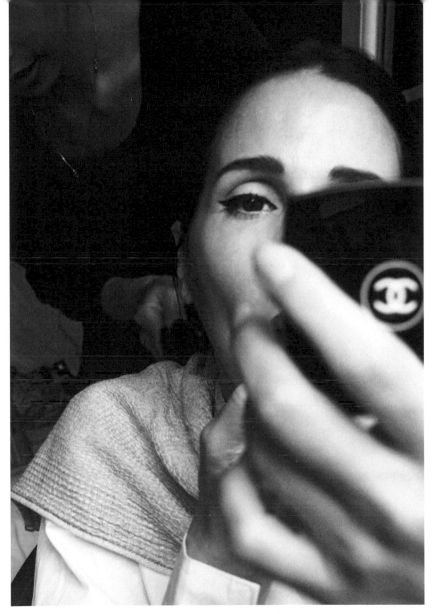

Muse/stylist Suzanne von Aichinger doing her make-up before
a video interview for Un Nouveau Ideal

Kingdom of Style

Michelle Haswell & Marie Thomson
kingdomofstyle.typepad.co.uk

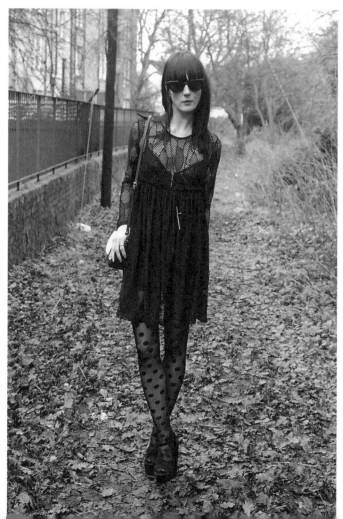

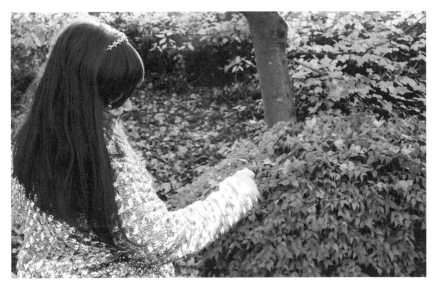

Above: Queen Marie
Opposite: Queen Michelle

Kingdom of Style is a relatively rare form of blog: one in which two creative minds come together equally to share their fashion and design inspirations. This is not a web magazine with two editors; it is a diary of personal aesthetic choices from two people whose stylistic tastes are aligned. Not initially conceived as something that would accrue a following of readers, their first posts were simply a way of working together on a project that allowed them an outlet for their fashion obsession. 'When we started, we were basically writing for and to each other. We didn't actually imagine that other people would find their way to the Kingdom', says Thomson. Six years later, Kingdom of Style has become the leading fashion blog to emerge from Scotland, nominated at both the Scottish Fashion Awards and the Scottish Style Awards. With a tougher, minimal yet elegantly feminine look in Thomson's case, or a more playful but defined one from Haswell, the duo juxtapose personal style posts with pieces on architecture, food - mostly cakes - and stories of their unique vintage discoveries.

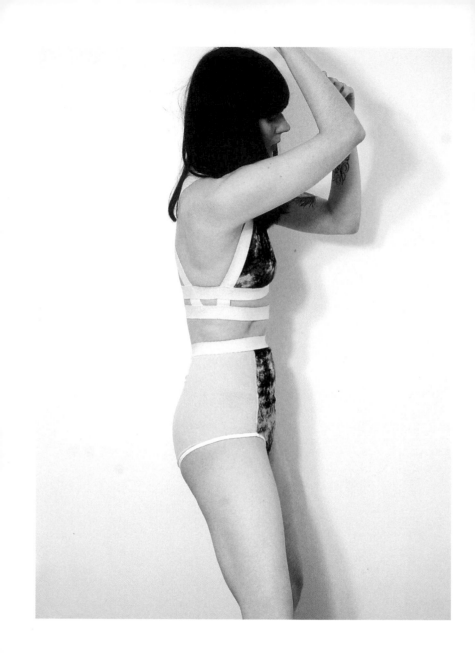

Michelle Haswell

'Marie was going through a tough time; we thought
starting a blog would not only be a good project
but also an ideal outlet for this passion we
shared. The blog was an online extension of our
real lives, in which we talked endlessly about
clothes and style.

While, like other bloggers, we do cover fashion,
the main difference is our age. We are coming from
the perspective of women in their thirties and
forties who don't conform to the expectations of
how women our age should dress. We are different
from other blogs not just in content but in tone.
Anecdotal, observational, outspoken and often
irreverent, we are free to feature whatever
is making our hearts race that day. If we look
at a trend or a designer's work and it provokes
emotion in us, then we want to write about it and
share it with others. Not just a designer, though;
it could just as easily be a song, a chair, a dress,
a handbag or even a movie. A good blog can provide
highly personal insights and a combination of
original and unique content which is regarded
by its readers as being more honest and truthful,
and is therefore more meaningful to them.'

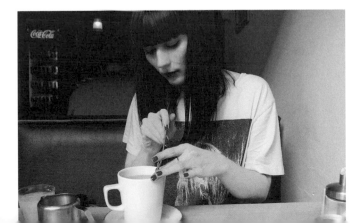

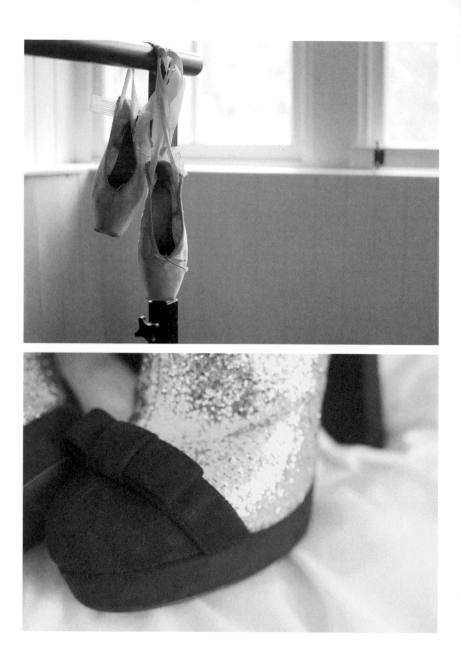

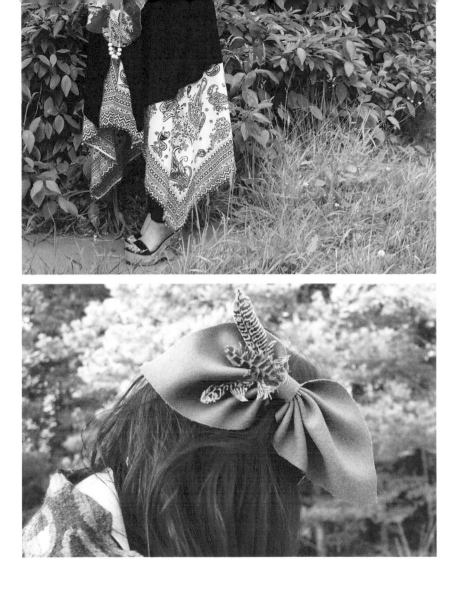

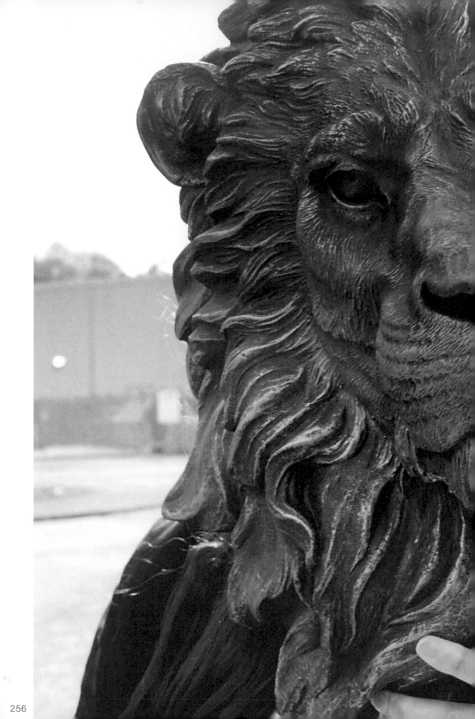

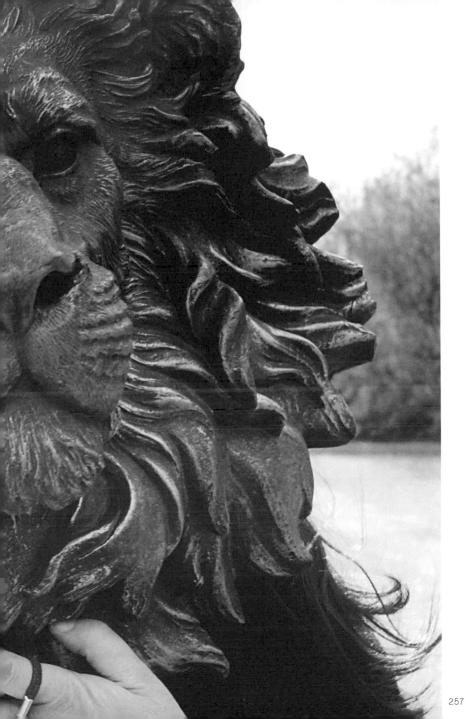

257

Face Hunter

Yvan Rodic

facehunter.org

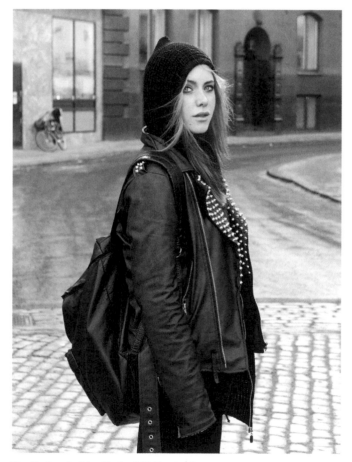

Stockholm - Fashion Week, A/W 12, day 1

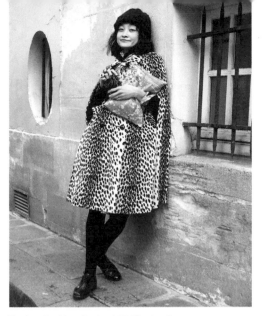

Paris - Fashion Week, A/W 12, day 6

Yvan Rodic's Face Hunter was one of the first street style photoblogs to emerge, capturing the essence of Parisians and the ways they dress. Now recognized as one of the leading blogs of its type, Face Hunter covers the individual styles of city-dwellers worldwide. Because of his work as an advertising copywriter and freelance writer, Rodic was well-versed in how to communicate messages clearly and combined this skill with his creative eye to create the blog. 'Blogging has changed my life. When I started it was just a little side project and now my blog is my main occupation. I get to travel all year long, publish books, realize campaigns for brands, direct fashion films, exhibit my photos and even guest design', he says. Rodic's aesthetic constantly changes; he is not interested in the latest trends but seeks to profile individuals who use the ways they dress to express their personalities. It is this attitude which carved out Rodic's niche and kept him an integral part of the blogosphere.

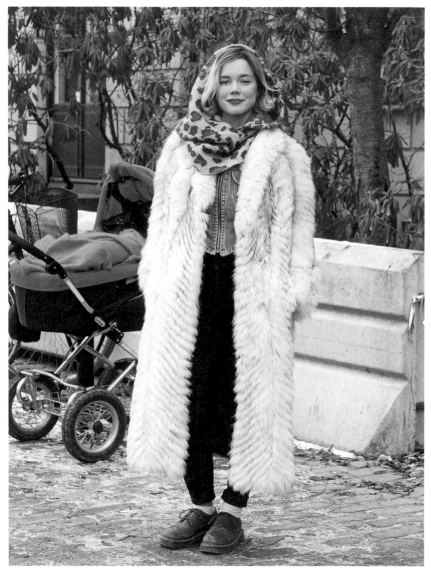

Stockholm – Fashion Week, A/W 12, day 3

Yvan Rodic

'When I moved from Switzerland to Paris,
I discovered a new world: fashion. My friends
would take me to shows and parties. I'd be so
excited about all the fabulous characters I'd meet
and felt I should share them with others. I like
to photograph people with a sense of individuality
who can combine elegance and creativity.

It's important to me to art direct my snapshots and
to spend time finding the appropriate background
to suit my subjects. I'm not interested in grouping
my photos into trends and putting them into boxes.
A trend for me is a repetition and that's a bit too
boring. I prefer to show a continuous flow of people
doing their own thing and let my reader decide what
they like; let them curate their own inspiration.

I celebrate individual style from all around the
world with an emphasis on "unusual" places such
as Kiev, Jakarta or Reykjavik, and don't only cover
the four big fashion weeks. Everybody already knows
about Paris or Milan; to me, posting an inspiring
picture from Santiago de Chile or Helsinki has
much more value.'

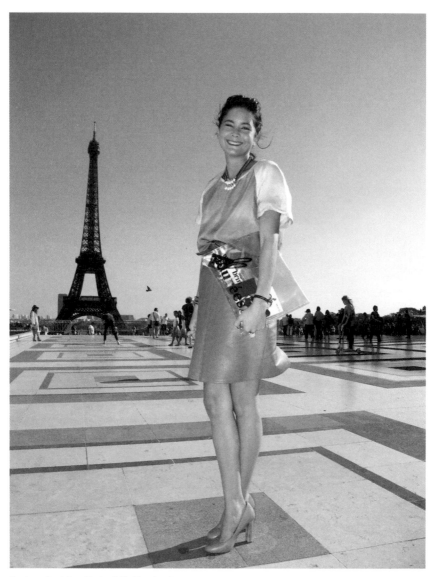

Paris – Fashion Week, S/S 12, day 2

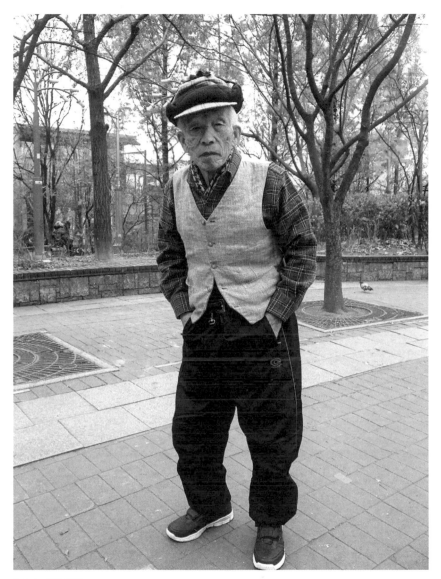

Seoul - Hongdae

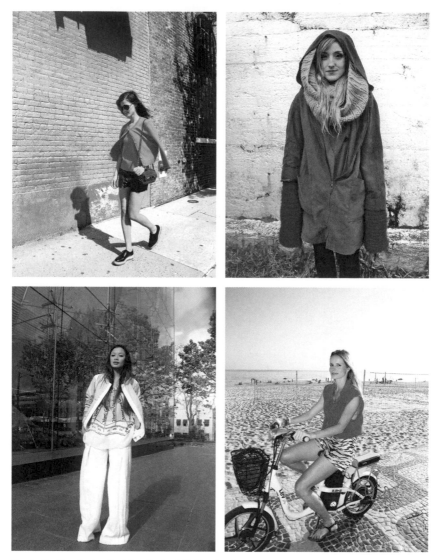

Top left: New York – Fashion Week, S/S 12, day 5
Top right: G! Festival – Gøta (Faroe Islands)
Bottom left: Sydney – Dannika, Bondi Beach
Bottom right: Rio de Janeiro – Carol, Ipanema

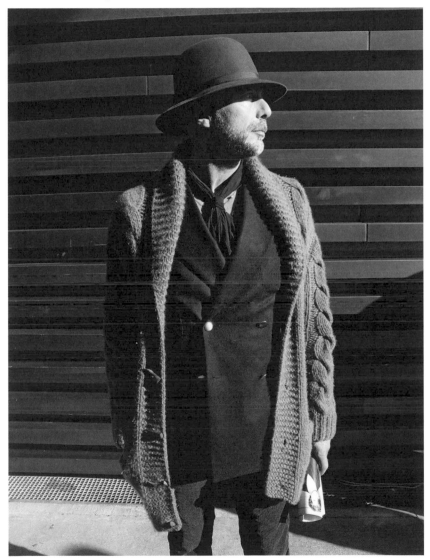

Garance Doré

Garance Doré

garancedore.fr

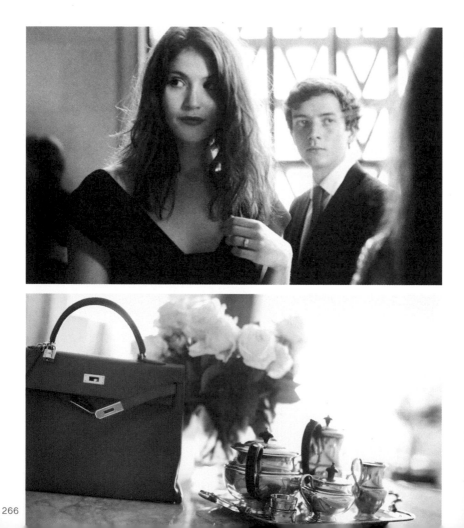

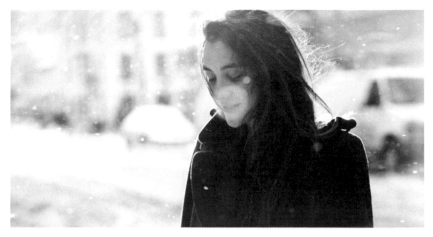

Above: Stevie Dance
Opposite top: Gemma Arterton
Opposite bottom: Kelly Bag by Hermès

Starting her career as an illustrator, Garance Doré set up
a blog in 2006 after becoming interested in what other people
were doing with the online platform. Her initial idea was
to gain direct feedback from readers on her art, but since
then both her practice and her readership have grown hugely.
Now known predominantly as a photographer with a distinctive
dreamlike and elegant style, Doré has become internationally
recognized, winning the 2012 CFDA Eugenia Sheppard Media Award
alongside her partner, The Sartorialist's Scott Schuman. After
meeting Schuman while still living in Paris, the couple moved
to New York, where Doré now works. She was described as 'possibly
the world's most closely followed blogger' by *Interview* magazine,
garnering around 50,000 hits a day. It is her eclectic yet well-
selected sets of images, thoughts and inspiration that keep her
avid audience returning. Doré provides style inspiration in her
own right, with her super-feminine, decisively French dress code.
She's been featured on the pages of *Elle* and the *New York Times*
among numerous other publications while maintaining a constant
presence on street style blogs the world over.

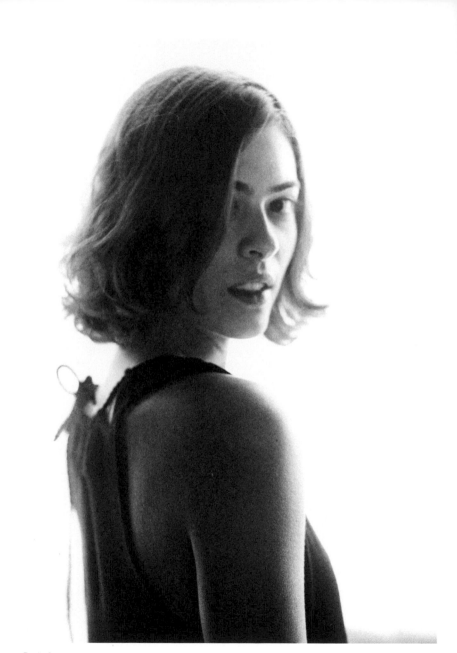

Isabel

Garance Doré

'I was working as an illustrator and growing
frustrated because I felt I wasn't connecting
with the readers of the magazines I was working
for. I had recently discovered blogs and decided
blogging could be a great way to get feedback
about my work. At first I just published a few
drawings, then I started adding text to my posts.
I found joy in sharing these snippets of my life
and engaging with my readers.

The blog has completely changed my life. It's
now my main occupation. As for my creativity,
it's a revolution to talk directly to an audience.
I listen to the feedback and I see what directly
touches people. I know how to understand the
difference between what's popular and what's
relevant. Most of the time it's the same, but
sometimes you have to make a bold decision
to talk about or show something that won't get
you praise from your audience. If I feel that
something is changing the trends or the way
we're seeing fashion, then I'm interested
in featuring it.

I think I have a very feminine point of view and
there is a softness in the way I see the world. I'm
not cynical or ironic, but I have a sense of humour
and of self-deprecation that adds perspective.
I always keep in mind that blogs were very personal
diaries when they started, and I try to keep up
that intimate conversation with my readers. Today
blogging is more integrated, less revolutionary.
I feel very happy to have been part of that shift.'

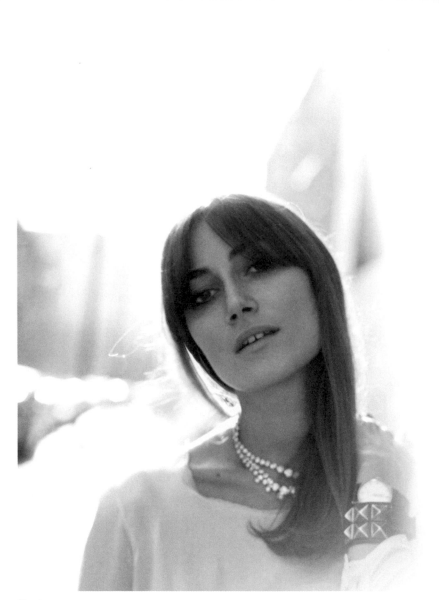

Gloria

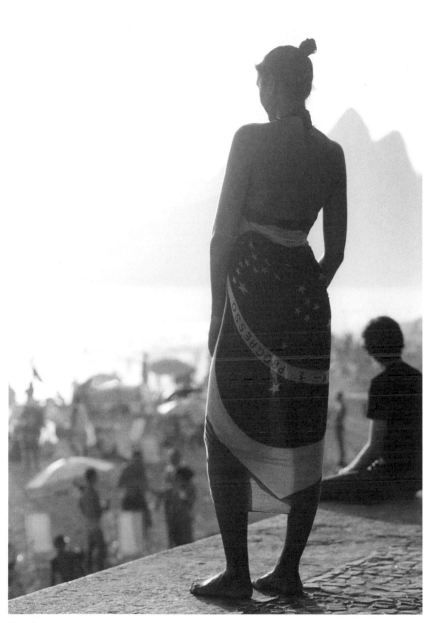

Rio, Ipanema

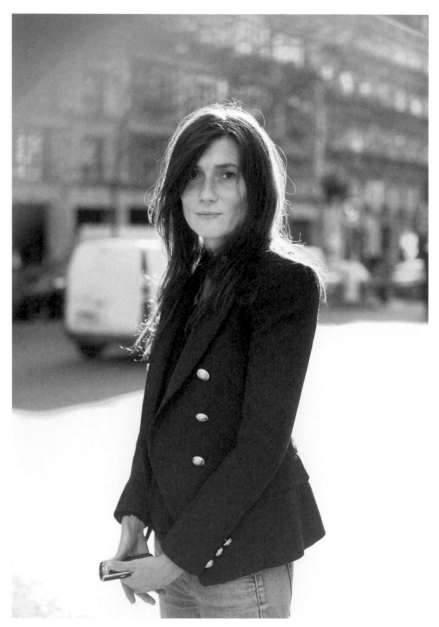

Emmanuelle Alt

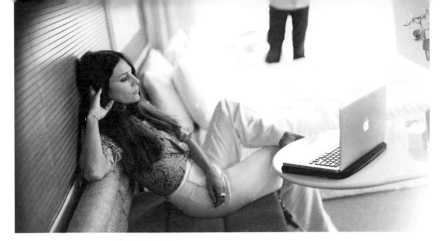

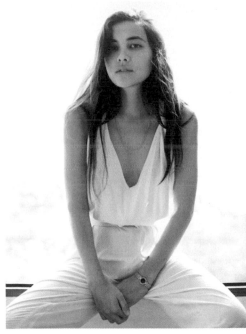

Top: Lisa Marie Fernandez, The Standard, New York
Bottom: Stevie Dance

StyleClicker

Gunnar Hämmerle

styleclicker.net

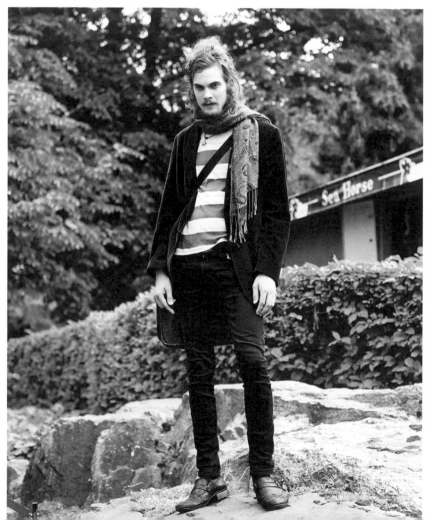

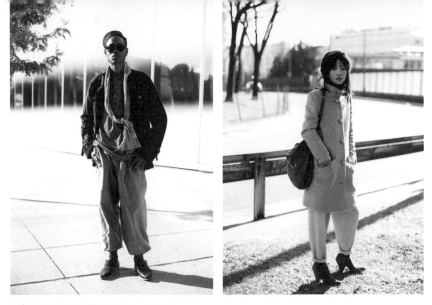

Left: New York - Mister Lee, editor
Right: Tender Tones, Paris - Miyuki, stylist
Opposite: On the Rocks, Helsinki - Jonathan, caretaker

After studying business management and subsequently running a small software firm with his brother, it was not until relatively late in his career that Gunnar Hämmerle started his site StyleClicker in 2006 from Germany. While looking to launch a portal that could be used as an online community, Hämmerle had the idea to focus on his own love of taking pictures. Now established as the leading German street style photoblog and one of the most viewed internationally, StyleClicker seeks out style as opposed to trends and high fashion, examining subjects for who they are as much as what they are wearing. Initially concentrating on his home town of Munich, Hämmerle now travels wordwide for the blog, shooting campaigns and editorials for Topman, Ben Sherman, German *Vogue*, GQ and *Vanity Fair*. Because Hämmerle comes from a non-industry background, his blog looks to dispel myths about fashion and open it up to everyone. 'Blogging has opened up the elite circle of fashion to common people, and it brought dialogue to the fashion world, where before there was only one-way communication', he explains.

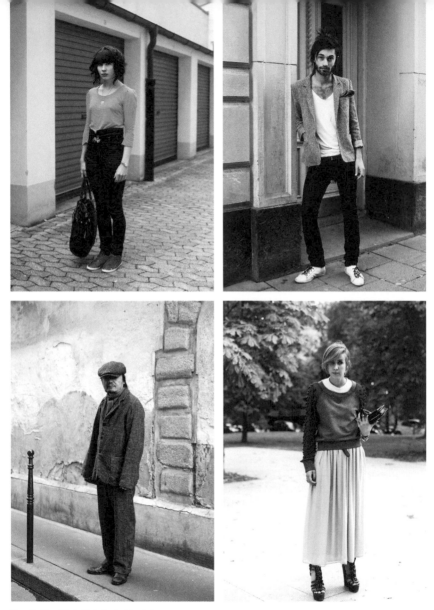

Top left: High Waisted, Munich
Top right: Cool Cuts, Stockholm
Bottom left: Painting, Paris – Hiroyuki, shop owner
Bottom right: Pretty in Pink, Milan – Simone, stylist

Gunnar Hämmerle

'I take portraits of interesting people, mainly
in the street, like studio shots but taken in
a natural environment. I guess the concept
is quite similar to any other street style blog.
The difference is how the concept is realized.
All the good street style blogs have their own
signature, their own aesthetics. I pick people
intuitively by following my subjective taste.
In the end, I am always interested in the people
I take pictures of; their style is just something
additional. I try to focus completely on my
subjects with no distraction from other things
happening around me. Lately I am finding fashion
weeks more and more annoying to shoot street
style at, always the same people and tons of
photographers shooting them, it's almost like
a war for the best picture.

I do not spend a lot of time visiting other
people's blogs. There are a few I check on a regular
basis but mostly because I know the people behind
them. The blog that probably influenced me most was
Hel Looks, great portraits always shot with the
same framing. As the aesthetics are always very
similar, there is no distraction from the
subject portrayed.'

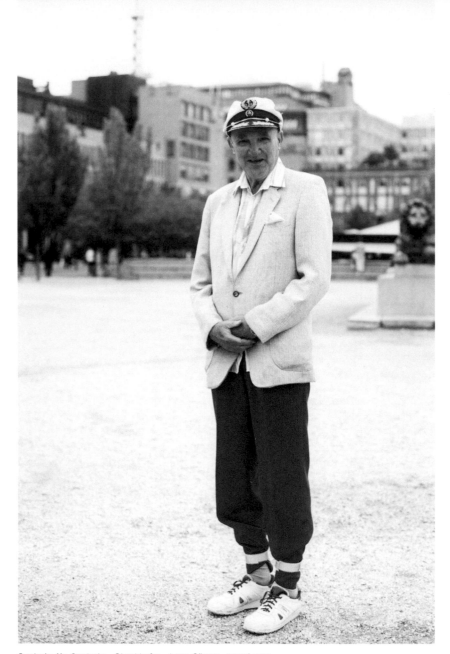

Captain My Captain, Stockholm - Lars Göran, pensioner

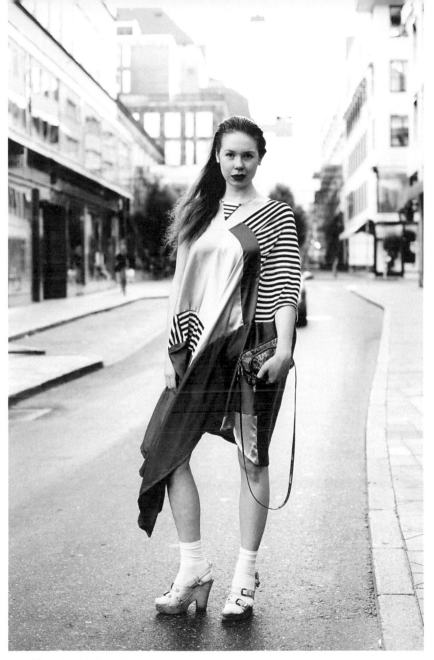

Into Blue, Stockholm - Yiva, designer

Stil in Berlin

Mary Scherpe & Dario Natale

stilinberlin.de

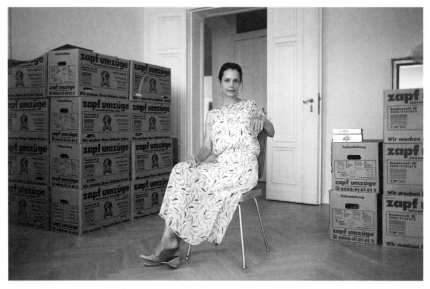

At home: Friederike Schilbach, editor at *Berlin Verlag*

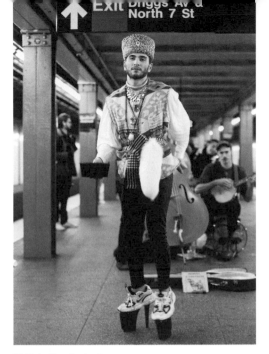

Stil in New York: Igor

Self-trained photographers Mary Scherpe and Dario Natale
decided to set up their Berlin street style photoblog in 2006.
Initially focusing on people they came across in their home
city and the outfits they wore, over time Stil in Berlin has
grown to cover a broader definition of style. As well as fashion,
their succinct, bright, graphic style of photography has been
turned to the worlds of film, food, music and the arts, covering
events, parties, people and places. Now Stil in Berlin is firmly
established as the German street style blog *du jour*. As the
blog's readership has grown, it has expanded into new forms
of coverage. What was once solely a photo-based site now
includes interviews with local artists, chefs and shop-owners
and portraits of people at home and at work, as well as guides
to Berlin and reports from fashion shows on young and
emerging designers.

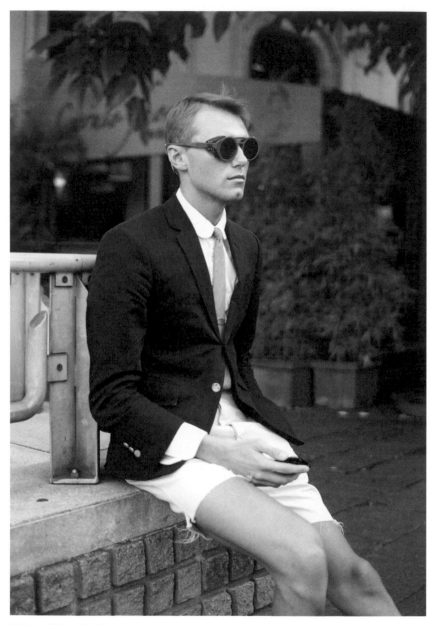

Stil in Milan: Matthew

Mary Scherpe & Dario Natale

'Blogging was the simplest, cheapest and quickest way to publish our version of Berlin fashion. Back in 2006, the international fashion blogging community was rather small and we felt very welcome.

We always look for a unique approach, a strong, self-confident appeal, for people with a refined sense of what they want to display through the clothing they create or wear. Part of our approach is to stay as open as possible, meaning we try not to define ourselves in order to avoid limitations. Of course, we can't deny our tastes: Mary is always drawn to menswear worn by women in a smart way; Dario to sleek, clean lines, often in black. Everything you see on Stil in Berlin is produced by us. We always aim for high-quality images and astute texts that go beyond what you can find on other blogs.'

Left: Stil in New York. Ekaterina
Right: Stil in Reykjavík: Eva

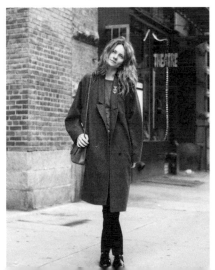 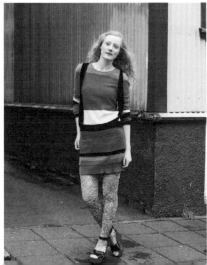

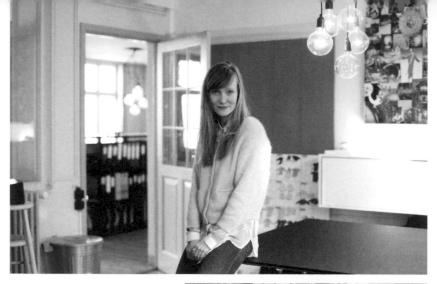

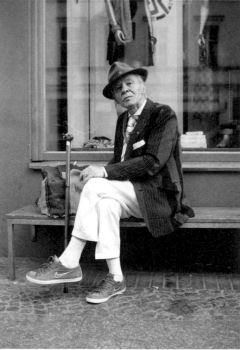

Top: At the studio: Stine Goya
Bottom: Stil in Berlin: Peter

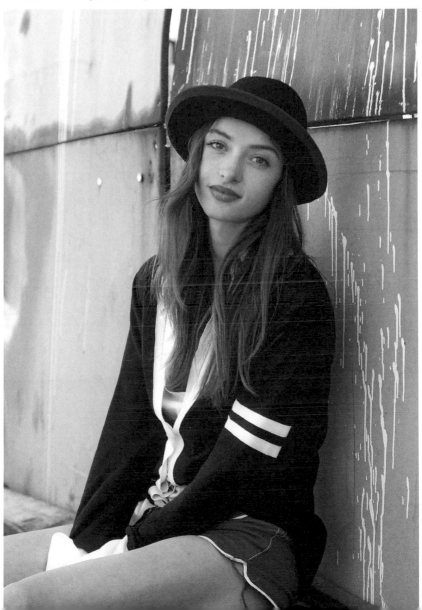

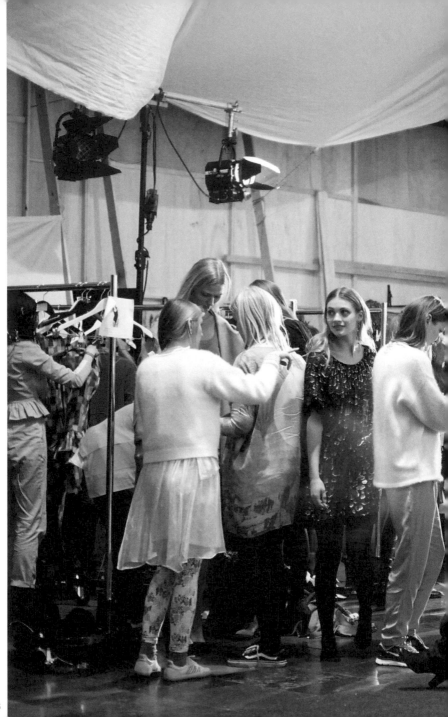

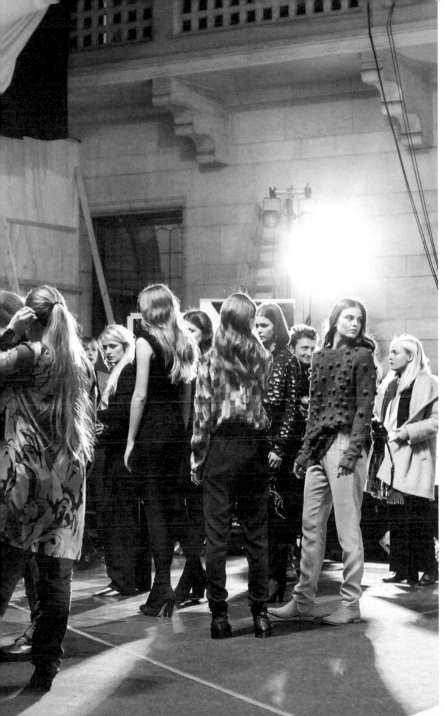

Street Peeper

Phil Oh

streetpeeper.com

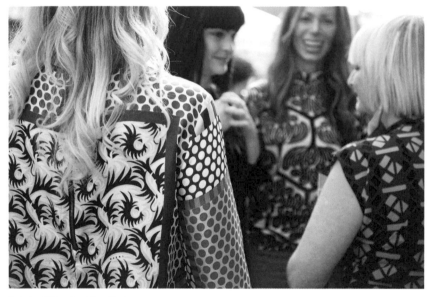

Print, Milan Fashion Week

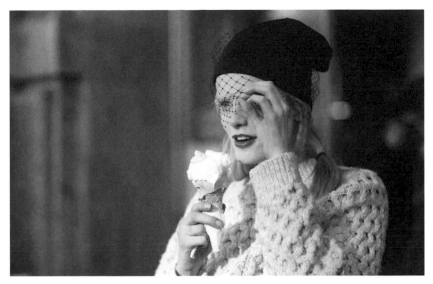

Hanne Gaby Odiele, Milan Fashion Week

Phil Oh earned a bachelor's degree in history from New York University, waited tables, created failed Internet start-ups and published a chick-lit novel, *Secrets of the Model Dorm*, before he started up his street style photoblog, Street Peeper, in 2006. Although clearly talented in a variety of fields, soon after launching the site in New York it became evident that capturing the world's most intriguing fashion looks was the 32-year-old's vocation. From the metropolises of Milan, Paris, London and New York to more obscure locations like Zurich, Oslo and Jakarta, Street Peeper provides eye-opening documentation of global style. Whether it's of famous editors, models and style icons or more unfamiliar faces, Oh's photography depicts a thoughtfully curated mix of eclectic and inspiring personal dress codes. Images range from spontaneous post-fashion-show snapshots to photos of the latest collections of design houses such as Lacoste and Helmut Lang. Aside from his own blog, Oh contributes to American Vogue.com, *Harper's Bazaar Australia* and *Elle China*, as well as working on campaigns for brands such as Saks Fifth Avenue.

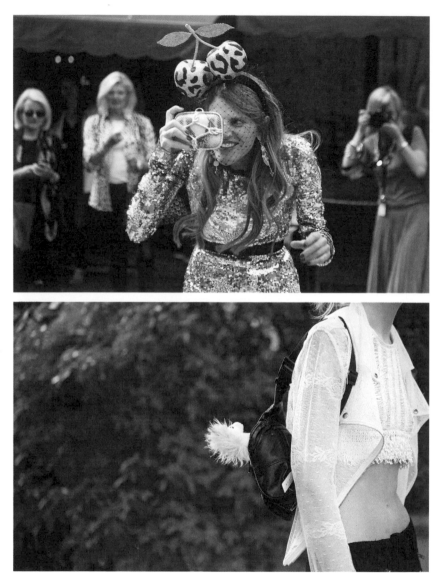

Top: Anna Dello Russo in Dolce & Gabbana, Milan Fashion Week
Bottom: Unicorns are real - London Fashion Week

Phil Oh

'When I first started blogging there weren't
a lot of street style blogs. The only ones I knew
of were The Sartorialist and Hel Looks. Face Hunter
had just started as well. I thought it would be fun
to go around taking pictures of people I viewed as
looking cool. Now my blog is my work and I've also
been commissioned through it.

I think blogging has brought an immediacy
to the fashion industry that didn't really exist
before. These days, I cover a lot more fashion
weeks and the subject-matter has also changed
in accordance with my interests and tastes. There
are so many blogs out there all attempting to do
similar things, so I suppose what differentiates
mine is simply my own personal point of view. I like
a lot of colour, print and pattern when done well,
which is rare. I don't really look for a particular
designer or trend, I just take pictures of things
that I like. If it happens to be a designer
or trend, then so be it.'

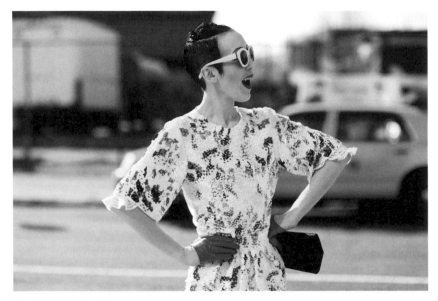

New York Fashion Week

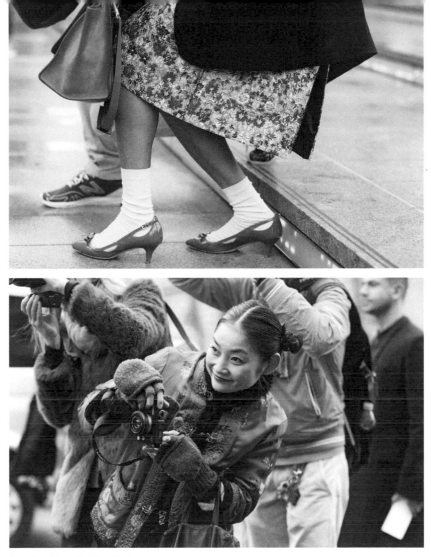

Top: New York Fashion Week
Bottom: Paris Fashion Week

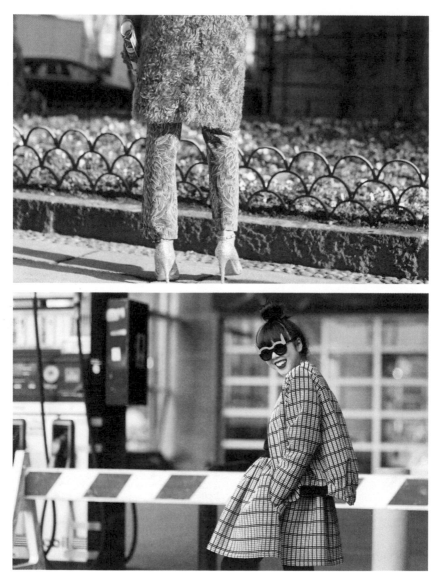

Top: Prada coat and Miu Miu heels, Milan Fashion Week
Bottom: Susie Bubble, New York Fashion Week

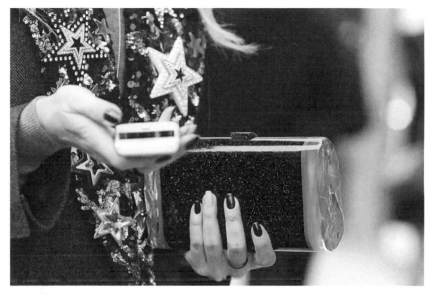

New York Fashion Week

Style Bubble

Susanna Lau

stylebubble.co.uk

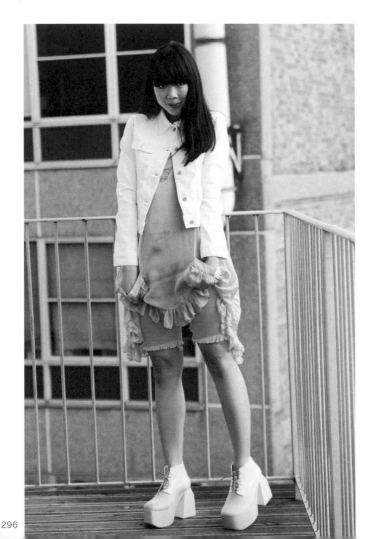

Susanna Lau, better known as the inimitable Susie Bubble,
author of the infectious blog Style Bubble, came to the world
of online publishing while studying history in 2006. Living
in London, surrounded by creativity and fashion, yet not truly
fulfilling her love for design through her coursework, developing
the blog allowed Lau an opportunity to delve inside the industry,
hunt out new talent and ultimately provide inspiration to her
now-devoted audience. Although at first a very personal outlet,
Style Bubble has rapidly grown in popularity, managing to touch
an army of readers from all corners of the globe. Recognized
for her talent in spotting and profiling upcoming names, in 2008
Lau was offered a role as editor of Dazed Digital, style magazine
Dazed & Confused's online platform. Style Bubble continued to
flourish throughout her time there and in 2011 Lau decided
to focus solely on her own vision. Since then Style Bubble has
become one of today's most revered and influential fashion blogs.
Subsequent collaborations have included Prada, Gap, Dr Martens
and Uniqlo and Lau is a regular contributor to print and online
publications including *The Observer*, *Vogue China*, *Elle UK* and
Pop magazine.

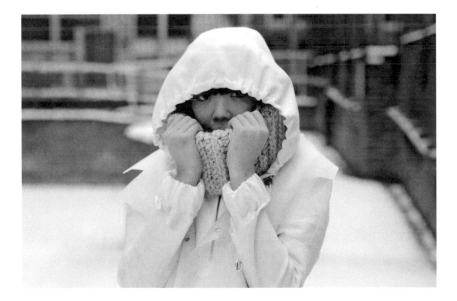

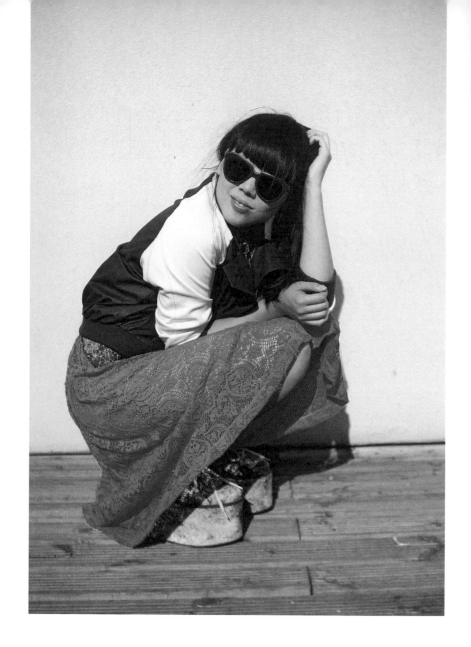

Susanna Lau

'I was working in quite a dull daytime job.
I wanted to take my interest in fashion to another
level, so a combination of sheer boredom and being
inspired by The Fashion Spot and a handful of blogs
spurred me on to get stuck in. It has always given
me a real buzz to create something that exists on
the Internet, so I guess the blog was a natural step
for me. I don't really think of the blog as work;
I'm always on the lookout for content and anything
can inspire a post. Feeding Style Bubble is very
much part of my daily routine.

The blog has given me opportunities to take on
work that I never thought I'd end up doing. This
has included styling, writing, editing and curating
on various levels. My schedule can be very hectic
and I travel a lot so I've had to adjust to that, but
I have no cause for complaint.

There is no one general aesthetic that I'm drawn
to. I like a unique point of view or designers
that really know what their identity is. I've
featured such an array of designers but I suppose
you could loosely call a lot of it "avant-garde"
design. I like a good story and an interesting
reference or inspiration point too - anything that
makes it easier for me to write about. It's always
important for me not just to show the imagery
of a designer but to explain what it is that draws
me to their work.'

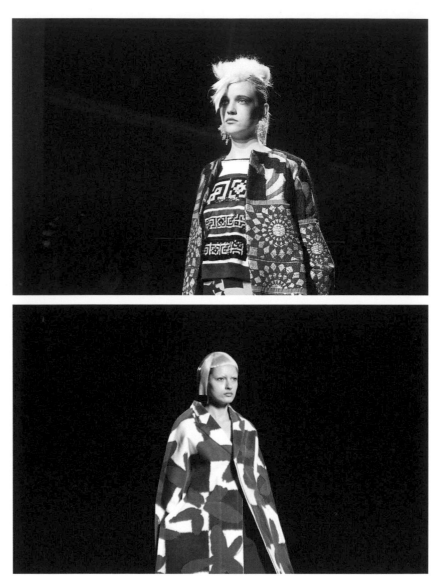

Top: Louise Gray, A/W 12, London Fashion Week
Bottom: Commes des Garçons, A/W 12

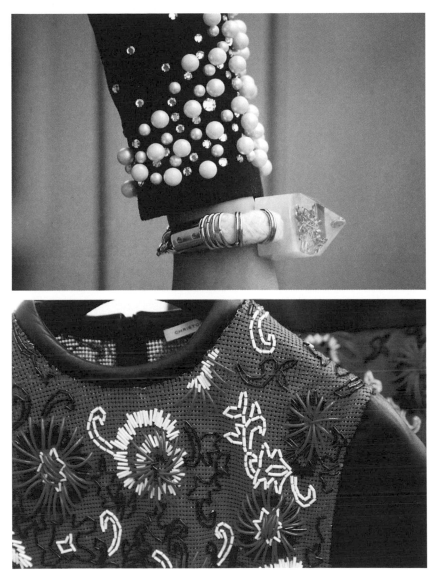

Bottom: Christopher Kane, from A/W 12 collection

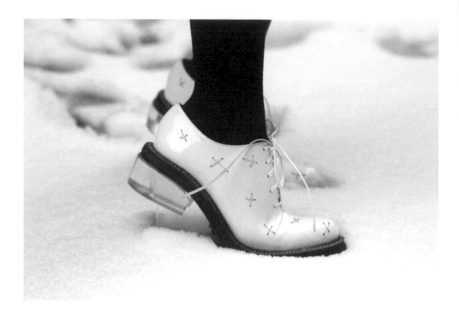

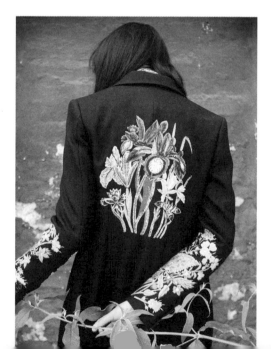

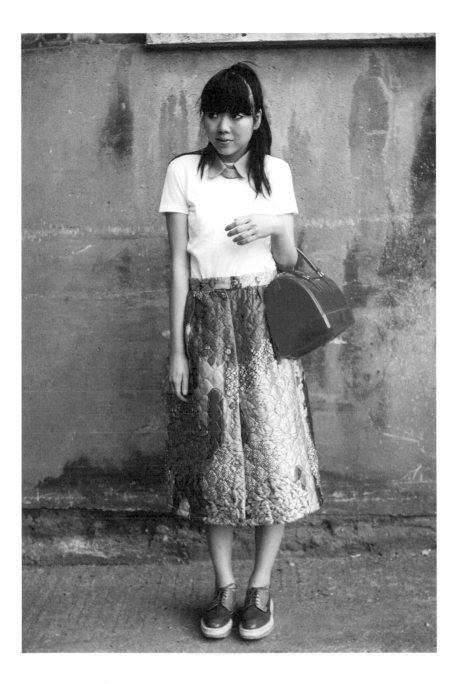

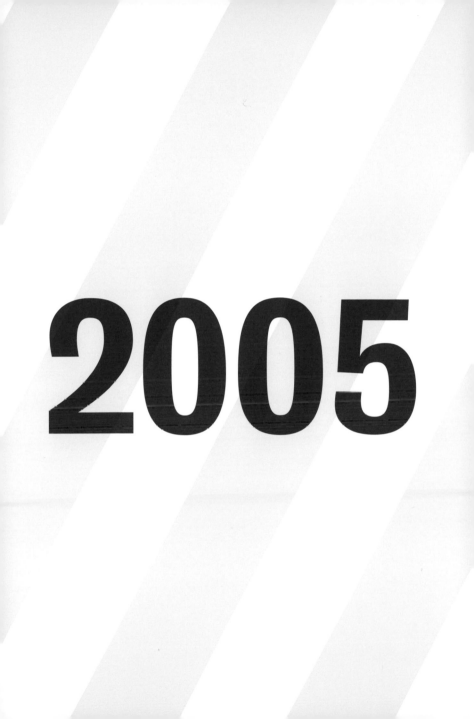

2005

Hypebeast

Kevin Ma

hypebeast.com

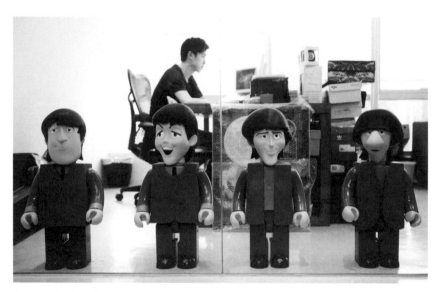

Kevin Ma in his office

After graduating with a double major in economics and psychology, Hong Kong-based Kevin Ma started his career in the finance sector before launching Hypebeast in 2005. The blog was initially a simple way for Ma to focus on his love of sneakers and streetwear. Rapidly collecting an eager following of readers worldwide, he soon quit his day job to dedicate his time to the site, gradually building it up to be one of the leading international digital portals for streetwear news. The site focuses on the obsessive collecting culture surrounding streetwear, reporting on new releases and collaborations from leading brands alongside profiles on emerging designers. Not solely centred on clothing, Hypebeast also looks at related forms of culture – graffiti, street and contemporary Pop art, music, design and photography – 'basically things that speak to us or will communicate with the Hypebeast person', says Ma. During the seven years the site has existed, streetwear culture has developed into a global commercial phenomenon. Hypebeast serves as both a testament to that phenomenon and a major supporting player in its continued success.

Essentials – Nooka founder Matthew Waldman

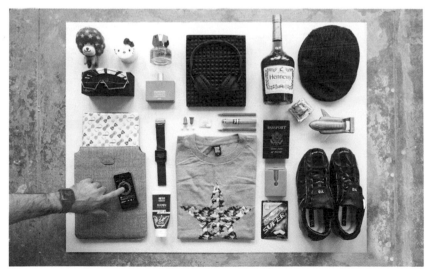

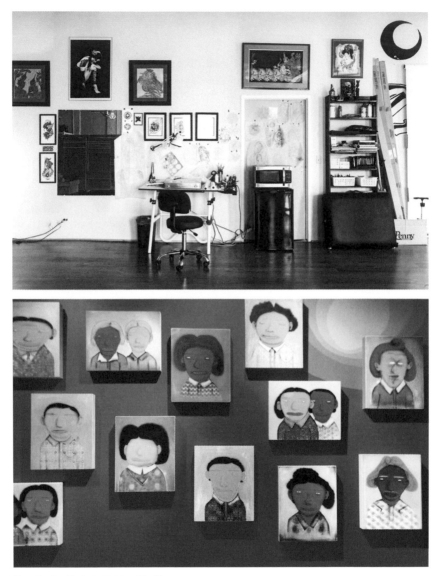

Top: Lucky Olelo's Tattoo Studio
Bottom: Os Gêmeos's 'Miss You' exhibition at Prism Gallery, Los Angeles

Kevin Ma

'I started blogging because I wanted a way to keep track of the things I liked and where to access them. Hypebeast has evolved through many stages. As time goes on, we're finding it is still growing and so are our readers, which provides us with the catalyst to continue searching for the unique and the unconventional. My aesthetic is pretty simple and clean, but the designers have to be innovative, fresh and new. We try to feature things that are one of a kind. We never try to be different but we always maintain our editorials and shape them to be informative. Fashion blogging provides quick access to information. The great thing about blogging is that it can be accessed anywhere and everywhere, by anyone in the world. It's free for people to enjoy, share and be inspired by.'

Shackman Store Renewal opening, Kobe, Japan

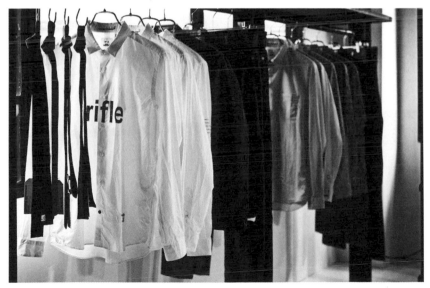

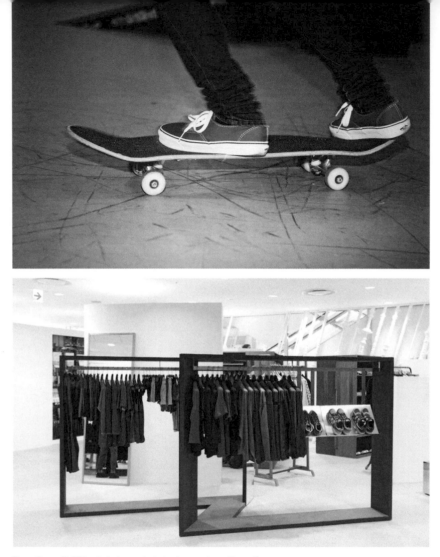

Top: Vans Sk85ive2 indoor skatepark opening, Hong Kong
Bottom: Dover St Market Ginza opening

Top: Essentials - DJ Jeff Solo
Bottom: Star Wars x Brisk Bodega Episode 0, Los Angeles

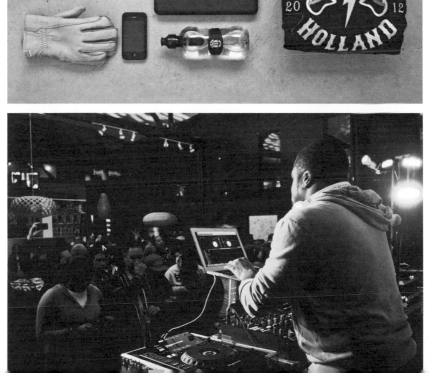

A Shaded View
on Fashion

Diane Pernet
ashadedviewonfashion.com

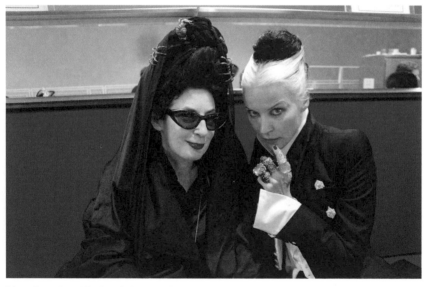

Diane Pernet and Daphne Guinness, Paris

Industry insider Diane Pernet, a fashion icon known for her often entirely black signature style, started A Shaded View on Fashion (ASVOF) from Paris back in 2005 when, as she recalls, 'Much of the world was still wondering, "What is blogging?"' ASVOF itself is mainly Pernet's visual diary of the people she meets, the places she goes and the things she sees. While her own voice is often kept to a minimum, Pernet reveals some of her inspirations through video and link posts focusing on music and art as well as fashion. Although now one of the blogging elite, she is equally well-known for her work across various different facets of the design world: as a former fashion designer and co-editor-in-chief of ZOO Magazine, and currently as a journalist for Elle.com and Vogueparis.com. Pernet also runs a leading fashion film festival, A Shaded View on Fashion Film, which launched in 2008 at the Jeu de Paume, Paris, and is now held annually at the Centre Pompidou.

Konstantinos Menelaou and Orian at the Charlie Le Mindu show

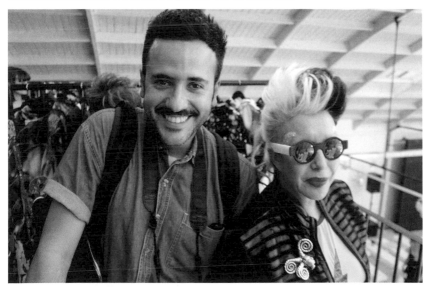

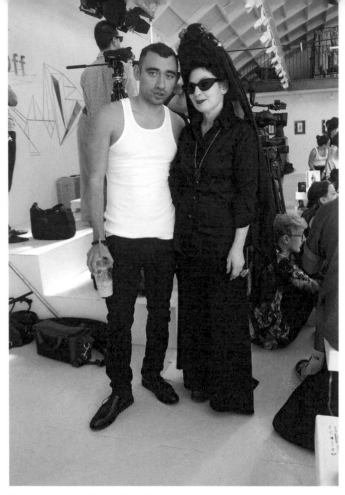

Nicola Formichetti and Diane Pernet backstage at the
Charlie Le Mindu show

Diane Pernet

'I couldn't care less about trends and have
always been of the belief that if you have to
follow trends, you are already too late. What
interests me is originality, people with their
own signature, like Rick Owens, Jean-Paul
Lespagnard, Haider Ackermann, musicians like
Woodkid, artists like Théo Mercier. Blogging
is a great platform for emerging as well as
established talent. I'm interested in the planet,
not just the major cities. Fashion is not the
only topic that interests me; my interests extend
into film, art, music, architecture, travel and
design, basically anything that I find creative
and inspiring. I suppose that via the blog people
have access to an intimate view of the world,
behind the ropes, so to speak. Aside from the
fact that at the beginning of the project I was
the only voice, it hasn't really changed since
I started. Now I find it more interesting having
a series of contributors, more than 20, who can
travel when I am not available, and whose style
of writing and vision corresponds with mine.'

The 'Diane' trophies for ASVOFF4, by Miguel Villalobos

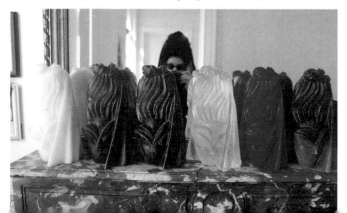

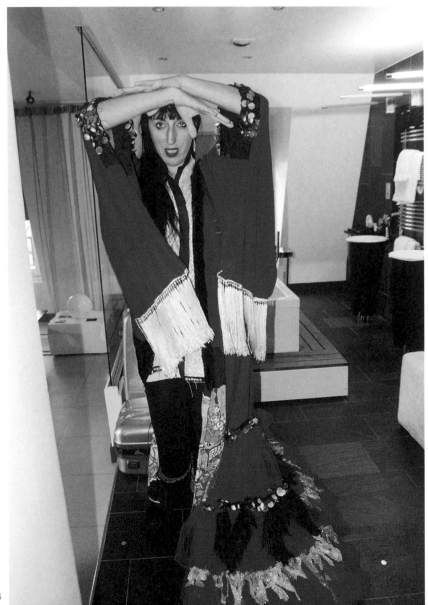

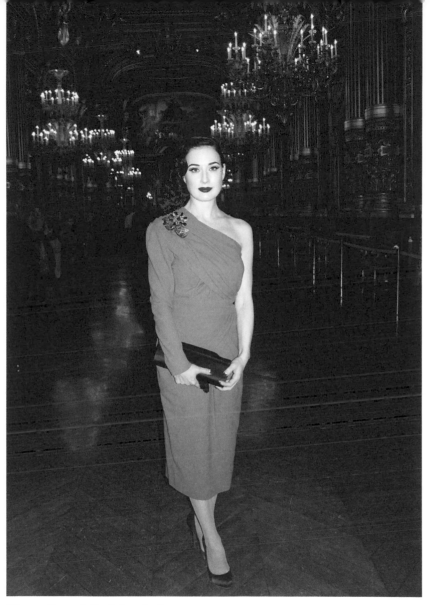

Dita von Teese at the Opéra, Paris

Acknowledgements

Thank you to all those involved in the project who gave their valuable time and advice, especially Susie Lau, Ali Gitlow, Carla Siepp, Andrew Hansen, Emma Clark, Federico Capalbo, Morgan Clement, Nick Shea, Martha Jay, Marianne Gunn O'Connor, Lara Angol and, for his enduring patience, Ryan Small.

William Oliver

I'd like to thank William Oliver for his patience and tenacity; all the bloggers who agreed to be featured, in particular my fellow food-loving street style snappers Phil Oh and Tommy Ton; and, last but not least, Steven Salter, for sticking with me.

Susanna Lau

Picture Credits

All photos © the individual bloggers, with the exception
of the following:

The Coveteur: ©Jake Rosenberg (pp.18-25); The Man Repeller:
©Naomi Shon (pp.28-35); Industrie: ©Rachel Chandler (pp.36-43);
Anna Dello Russo: ©Giampaolo Sgura (pp.44, 46), ©Scott Schuman
(p.48), ©Inez van Lamsweerde (p.49 top), ©Shoot the Breeze
(p.49 bottom left); Patternity: ©Georges Antoni (p.68 top);
What Katie Wore: ©Joe Sinclair (pp.88-95); Cocorosa: ©Ilanka
Verhoeven (p.97), ©Suzanne Ford-Carafano (p.98); Advanced Style:
©Jenna Dublin (p.113); Lulu and Your Mom: ©Timothy Petersen
(pp.132-37); Disneyrollergirl: ©David Hill (p.190 top);
The Business of Fashion: ©Daniel Cianfarra (p.204), ©Victor
Virgile (p.205), ©Morgan O'Donovan (p.206 top), ©Handout
(p.206 bottom), ©Timothy A. Clary (p.208 top), ©Eric Ryan
(p.208 bottom), ©Dustin Fenstermacher (p.209); Fashionista:
©Ashley Jahncke (pp.210-17); Amlul: ©Zoe Noble (pp.218-19),
©Sam Butt (pp.220, 222, 224-25), ©Saga Sig (p.221), ©Tinko
Czetwertynski (p.223); Selectism: ©Ross Trevail (pp.234-39);
Stil in Berlin: ©Mary Scherpe (pp.278, 281-83),
©Dario Natale (pp.279-80, 284-85).

Cover: top ⊕Susanna Lau, Style Bubble
(see page 296); centre ⊕Jayne Min,
Stop It Right Now (see page 82); bottom
⊕Tommy Ton, Jak & Jil (see page 124)

Back cover: ⊕David Hill,
Disneyrollergirl (see page 188)

Prestel, A member of Verlagsgruppe
Random House GmbH

Prestel Verlag
Neumarkter Str. 28
81673 Munich
Tel. +49 (0)89 4136-0
Fax +49 (0)89 4136-2335
www.prestel.de

Prestel Publishing Ltd.
4 Bloomsbury Place
London WC1A 2QA
Tel. +44 (0)20 7323-5004
Fax +44 (0)20 7636-8004
www.prestel.com

Prestel Publishing
900 Broadway, Suite 603
New York, NY 10003
Tel. +1 (212) 995-2720
Fax +1 (212) 995-2733
www.prestel.com

Library of Congress Control Number:
2012939410

British Library Cataloguing-in-
Publication Data: a catalogue record
for this book is available from the
British Library.

The Deutsche Nationalbibliothek holds
a record of this publication in the
Deutsche Nationalbibliografie; detailed
bibliographical data can be found under:
http://dnb.d-nb.de

Prestel books are available worldwide.
Please contact your nearest bookseller
or one of the above addresses for
information concerning your local
distributor.

Editorial direction: Ali Gitlow
Editorial assistance: Carla Siepp
Editorial interns: Katie Balcombe,
Francesca Dunnett
Copyedited by: Martha Jay
Production: Friederike Schirge
Design and layout: Praline

Origination: Reproline Mediateam, Munich
Printing and binding: Druckerei Uhl GmbH &
Co. KG, Radolfzell
Printed in Germany

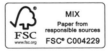

MIX
Paper from
responsible sources
FSC
www.fsc.org
FSC® C004229

Verlagsgruppe Random House FSC-DEU-0100
The FSC-certified paper Tauro has been
supplied by Papier Union, Germany
ISBN 978-3-7913-4718-9